Neck Pain

Neck Pain Treatment & Exercise Solutions

(How to Perform Neck–exercises for Neck Pain and Shoulder Pain Relief)

Devin Ryan

Published By **Phil Dawson**

Devin Ryan

All Rights Reserved

Neck Pain: Neck Pain Treatment & Exercise Solutions (How to Perform Neck–exercises for Neck Pain and Shoulder Pain Relief)

ISBN   978-1-9992826-9-1

Legal & Disclaimer

Table Of Contents

Chapter 1: The Importance Of Accurate Diagnosis

Identifying the Root Cause for Targeted Treatment

The accurate evaluation of neck pain is critical for offering effective and centered treatment to sufferers. Neck ache, a commonplace situation that influences a huge percent of the populace, should have numerous underlying motives. These motives can range from easy muscle lines to more complicated problems like degenerative situations, nerve compression, and trauma. By figuring out the idea purpose, healthcare companies can tailor remedy alternatives that address the underlying trouble, decrease the risk of recurrence, and sell prolonged-time period comfort for patients.

Muscle strain is one of the most commonplace motives of neck ache, regularly because of overuse, terrible posture, or slumbering in a clumsy position. When the neck muscle groups are strained or overworked, they may be able to emerge as infected and painful, maximum essential to decreased mobility and pain. Identifying muscle strain as the basis motive of neck pain lets in healthcare carriers to indicate suitable remedies, including relaxation, ice, warmth, gentle stretching, and over the counter pain relievers.

Poor posture can also make a contribution notably to neck ache. The prolonged use of digital gadgets, sitting at a desk for extended periods, and distinctive life-style elements can cause wrong alignment of the cervical backbone, setting excessive strain at the neck muscle organizations and ligaments. Identifying terrible posture due to the fact the underlying cause of neck ache lets in healthcare providers to propose ergonomic modifications, postural sporting sports activities, and bodily treatment to alleviate pain and sell better posture.

Degenerative situations, alongside aspect cervical spondylosis or degenerative disc illness, also can purpose neck ache. These conditions contain the sluggish deterioration of the intervertebral discs, side joints, and other systems within the cervical spine, main to stiffness, inflammation, and possibly nerve compression. When healthcare businesses come to be privy to a degenerative scenario as the basis purpose of neck ache, treatment options can also additionally encompass remedy, bodily treatment, and in extra intense instances, surgical intervention.

Nerve compression is another commonplace reason of neck pain, frequently supplying as radicular ache that radiates down the arm. This can quit result from a herniated disc, spinal stenosis, or foraminal stenosis, which can compress or worsen the cervical nerve roots. Identifying nerve compression because of the truth the motive of neck ache permits healthcare providers to suggest targeted treatments, together with epidural steroid injections, nerve blocks, or surgical decompression, relying on the severity and length of the circumstance.

Trauma, which embody whiplash or a proper away impact to the cervical backbone, can also bring about neck ache. Injuries may additionally incorporate damage to the muscle corporations, ligaments, aspect joints, or intervertebral discs, vital to infection, instability, and possibly neurological symptoms and symptoms and signs and signs and symptoms. When healthcare vendors choose out trauma as the idea cause of neck ache, remedy alternatives may also additionally involve a aggregate of conservative measures, which includes rest, immobilization, and treatment, as well as more competitive interventions like surgical treatment or rehabilitation, relying at the severity of the damage and the affected person's individual desires.

Accurately identifying the muse purpose of neck ache is important for offering focused and effective remedy. By carefully thinking

4

about the affected character's information, signs and symptoms, and diagnostic findings, healthcare providers can tailor remedy plans that deal with the underlying trouble, lower the threat of recurrence, and promote long-term consolation for patients affected by neck ache.

A complete information of the neck's anatomy is essential for correct analysis and remedy of neck ache. The cervical spine, or neck, is a complex form together with bones, joints, muscles, ligaments, tendons, and nerves that artwork collectively to assist the pinnacle and allow a big kind of motion.

The cervical backbone is created from seven vertebrae, classified C1 via C7. The first vertebrae, C1 (atlas) and C2 (axis), are specific of their form and function, taking into consideration the pivotal moves of the top, which includes nodding and rotation. The last cervical vertebrae, C3 to C7, are greater similar in shape and facilitate the neck's flexion, extension, and lateral bending.

Between each pair of vertebrae, intervertebral discs offer cushioning and guide, absorbing marvel and bearing in mind flexibility. Each disc includes a mild, gel-like middle known as the nucleus pulposus, surrounded with the aid of the use of a extra difficult, fibrous outer layer known as the annulus fibrosus. Over time, those discs may additionally additionally enjoy degenerative changes or harm, in all likelihood leading to conditions in conjunction with herniated or bulging discs.

The spinal canal runs thru the center of the cervical vertebrae, housing and protective the spinal cord. The spinal cord is a essential a part of the applicable frightened gadget, transmitting data the various mind and the relaxation of the body. At every degree of the cervical backbone, pairs of spinal nerves branch off from the spinal cord and exit via small openings called intervertebral foramina. These cervical nerves are chargeable for controlling sensation and movement inside the neck, shoulders, fingers, and arms.

Compression or contamination of those nerves can result in neck pain, in addition to radiating ache or neurological symptoms inside the top extremities.

Various muscle organizations, ligaments, and tendons in the neck vicinity offer stability, help, and facilitate motion. The muscle tissue of the neck are typically classified into 3 groups: superficial, intermediate, and deep. The superficial muscle corporations, together with the sternocleidomastoid and trapezius, are via and huge answerable for large moves along side head rotation and neck extension. The intermediate and deep muscles, which include the scalenes and the suboccipital muscle mass, provide more specific movements and assist maintain proper alignment of the cervical vertebrae.

Ligaments, which might be strong bands of connective tissue, be part of the cervical vertebrae and help stabilize the spine. Key ligaments inside the neck embody the anterior and posterior longitudinal ligaments, which run alongside the front and back of the vertebral our our bodies, and the ligamentum flavum, which connects the laminae of adjoining vertebrae. Tendons, some different type of connective tissue, join muscle groups to bones, thinking about the switch of stress and motion.

The anatomy of the neck is a complex and interconnected device of bones, joints, muscle groups, ligaments, tendons, and nerves that artwork together to help the top and permit a large variety of movement. A thorough records of those systems and their capabilities is essential for correct prognosis and remedy of neck pain.

An accurate prognosis of neck pain starts offevolved offevolved with a entire affected man or woman facts and physical exam. Obtaining an in depth affected man or woman history is vital to understand the context in which neck ache happens and end up privy to viable contributing factors. During the facts-taking approach, healthcare companies acquire facts at the onset, period, severity, and area of pain. They additionally inquire approximately any associated symptoms and signs and symptoms, together with numbness or tingling in the higher extremities, complications, or trouble drowsing.

The affected person's clinical records performs a massive function within the diagnostic device. Healthcare providers remember previous accidents, surgical strategies, and comorbidities that would make contributions to neck pain or predispose the affected character to unique conditions. For instance, a facts of rheumatoid arthritis may additionally moreover suggest an inflammatory purpose for neck pain, whilst a previous motor vehicle twist of fate also can beautify suspicion of whiplash-related problems. Furthermore, a evaluate of medicinal capsules, hypersensitive reactions, and way of lifestyles elements, together with profession and physical hobby degrees, can offer more insights into functionality reasons and danger elements for neck ache.

During the bodily examination, the healthcare issuer assesses the affected person's posture, paying near interest to any signs and symptoms and signs of ahead head posture, rounded shoulders, or different misalignments which can make a contribution to neck strain. The affected person's style of motion is evaluated, with the healthcare provider guiding the affected person via numerous neck moves, which includes flexion, extension, lateral flexion, and rotation, to understand any barriers or ache provocation.

Muscle electricity and reflexes are assessed to evaluate the ability involvement of the cervical nerves. The healthcare company can also moreover take a look at the power of the affected individual's neck, shoulder, and arm muscles and take a look at reflexes at unique factors, at the aspect of the biceps, triceps, and brachioradialis. Any asymmetry or deficits in strength or reflexes can provide clues about capability nerve involvement.

Special checks, including the Spurling take a look at, may be completed to recognize nerve root compression. In the Spurling test, the affected character's head is lightly prolonged and turned around toward the symptomatic side, and a downward pressure is completed to the pinnacle of the pinnacle. The test is considered exceptional if it reproduces the affected person's arm ache or neurological signs and signs, suggesting nerve root compression.

Palpation of the neck and shoulder muscle corporations can assist choose out out muscle pressure, cause elements, or localized contamination. The healthcare employer gently presses on numerous muscle corporations, together with the trapezius, levator scapulae, and sternocleidomastoid, to evaluate for tenderness or tightness. Palpation also can display joint tenderness, which might probably endorse arthritis or one-of-a-kind joint-associated troubles.

In some times, more assessments can be vital to rule out extraordinary capability causes of neck ache. For example, a radical examination of the temporomandibular joint (TMJ) can assist end up privy to TMJ sickness as a contributing detail. Similarly, an evaluation of the shoulder joint and surrounding structures can assist determine if the neck pain is referred from the shoulder or if each regions are independently affected.

Overall, a whole affected man or woman records and bodily examination are crucial additives of the diagnostic manner for neck ache. By carefully considering the affected character's symptoms and signs and symptoms and signs and symptoms, medical records, and bodily findings, healthcare agencies can growth a going for walks speculation of the underlying cause and direct in addition diagnostic tests and remedy therefore.

Imaging studies play a essential position in the diagnostic technique for neck pain, as they permit healthcare organizations to visualise the inner systems of the cervical spine and surrounding tissues. These imaging techniques can screen the presence of fractures, dislocations, degenerative adjustments, and different abnormalities that can be contributing to neck pain.

One of the maximum commonplace imaging techniques used inside the evaluation of neck ache is the X-ray. This form of imaging makes use of a small amount of ionizing radiation to create photographs of the bony structures in the cervical backbone. X-rays can help healthcare providers discover fractures or dislocations, which may also additionally rise up because of trauma or damage. Additionally, X-rays can display degenerative changes within the cervical backbone, which incorporates the presence of arthritis or osteophyte (bone spur) formation. These degenerative modifications can cause joint irritation, reduced range of movement, and nerve compression, principal to neck pain and other signs and symptoms. While X-rays are a precious device inside the assessment of neck ache, they do now not provide distinct pix of smooth tissues, together with muscle groups, ligaments, and intervertebral discs.

It is critical to note that despite the fact that X-rays are a significantly used diagnostic device, in addition they have barriers. X-ray images can every so often be difficult to interpret due to overlapping systems, and they will now not seize diffused abnormalities or early-degree degenerative adjustments. As a result, greater imaging research can be important to accumulate a extra entire know-how of the underlying reason of neck ache.

Magnetic Resonance Imaging (MRI) is a powerful diagnostic device that offers precise snap shots of the cervical spine, consisting of the smooth tissues together with muscle agencies, ligaments, and intervertebral discs. It has end up a beneficial tool for healthcare professionals in the exceptional assessment of neck pain, because it lets in for the visualization of systems that cannot be seen with traditional X-rays or CT scans.

MRI works with the useful resource of the usage of a mixture of a robust magnetic concern, radio waves, and a computer to generate excessive-desire snap shots of the inner systems of the body. During the MRI test, the affected character lies down on a movable table that slides into the MRI system, which is largely a massive, cylindrical magnet. The magnetic difficulty aligns the hydrogen atoms inside the body, and whilst radio waves are executed, the hydrogen atoms absorb after which release power, generating signals that the MRI machine detects and uses to create images.

One of the number one blessings of MRI in the analysis of neck ache is its ability to visualise gentle tissues, it simply is specifically beneficial for figuring out disc herniation. A herniated disc, every now and then referred to as a slipped or ruptured disc, takes region while the clean internal center of an intervertebral disc protrudes through the outer fibrous layer. This can motive stress on close by nerves or the spinal wire, most important to pain, numbness, and weak spot within the neck, shoulder, or arm. MRI can show the size, area, and quantity of disc herniation, providing valuable information for making plans appropriate treatment strategies.

MRI is also pretty powerful in diagnosing spinal stenosis, a situation in which the spinal canal narrows, potentially compressing the spinal twine or nerve roots. Spinal stenosis can give up result from a selection of things, which include degenerative changes, bone spurs, or disc herniation. MRI can visualize the narrowing of the spinal canal, further to any associated smooth tissue abnormalities, which encompass thickened ligaments or bulging discs, that may be contributing to the compression.

Spinal cord compression, or myelopathy, is a few exclusive important circumstance that MRI can assist grow to be privy to. Myelopathy could have severa reasons, together with spinal stenosis, disc herniation, or tumors, and may reason enormous neurological signs if left untreated. MRI provides an awesome view of the spinal cord, permitting healthcare professionals to evaluate the quantity of compression, turn out to be privy to the motive, and plan for appropriate interventions, including surgical operation or conservative management.

In addition to those unique conditions, MRI moreover may be used to diagnose different motives of neck ache, which includes ligament accidents, muscle traces, and infections, or to rule out extra vital conditions like tumors. Overall, the functionality of MRI to provide particular pics of the cervical backbone and its surrounding systems makes it an critical device inside the correct diagnosis and control of neck pain.

A computed tomography (CT) check is a complicated imaging approach that uses X-rays and computer technology to create distinct skip-sectional pictures, or "slices," of the cervical spine. By compiling these slices, a CT take a look at provides a whole view of the bony systems inside the neck, permitting healthcare companies to assess the cervical backbone's common state of affairs.

One of the principle benefits of a CT take a look at over preferred X-rays is its functionality to supply extra exact photos of the bony systems within the cervical backbone. This better decision permits healthcare groups to select out diffused fractures, degenerative changes, and bone spurs greater because it have to be. Furthermore, a CT check can offer extra records at the alignment and stability of the cervical backbone, which may be critical in times of trauma or suspected instability.

Chapter 2: Conservative Treatment Approaches

Non-Invasive Methods to Alleviate Neck Pain

Conservative treatment strategies for neck pain usually attention on non-invasive techniques to relieve pain, decorate feature, and sell recovery. These strategies are designed to govern pain and repair the neck's normal variety of movement without resorting to surgical intervention. Neck pain can prevent end result from diverse motives, collectively with muscle pressure, ligament sprains, joint disorder, nerve compression, and degenerative adjustments in the cervical backbone. Identifying the underlying reason of neck ache is essential for choosing the maximum suitable conservative treatment method and optimizing consequences.

One of the maximum common conservative remedy strategies for neck pain is pain treatment. Both over-the-counter and prescription medications can help manipulate ache and inflammation, supplying transient consolation and permitting the man or woman to interact in exceptional rehabilitative treatment options. Pain treatment is regularly used on the issue of various conservative remedies, collectively with physical treatment, to address the foundation reason of neck pain and sell lengthy-time period restoration.

Physical remedy is each exclusive cornerstone of conservative neck ache remedy. A complete physical treatment software can assist to beautify neck mobility, muscle power, and staying electricity, addressing muscle imbalances and joint sickness contributing to neck ache. Physical treatment for neck pain regularly includes a mixture of manual remedy strategies, healing carrying activities, and modalities, which includes warmth and bloodless therapy or electric powered stimulation. By targeted at the precise impairments and limitations of the person, physical treatment can assist to relieve neck pain and prevent its recurrence.

Heat and bloodless therapy are widely used conservative treatment strategies for handling neck ache, as they offer resultseasily available and espresso-fee options for ache comfort. By alternating the software of warmth and cold to the affected vicinity, people can lessen inflammation, muscle tension, and pain. Understanding the precise signs and symptoms and signs and symptoms and contraindications for heat and cold treatment, as well as the proper application techniques, is essential for maximizing their therapeutic advantages.

Ergonomic changes, which include posture correction and modifications to the person's paintings and sleep environments, can play a essential feature in the conservative management of neck pain. Poor posture and wrong ergonomics can vicinity excessive pressure at the cervical backbone and surrounding muscle groups, contributing to neck ache and sickness. By making centered adjustments to the man or woman's every day conduct and surroundings, ergonomic interventions can help to reduce neck pain and sell prolonged-term musculoskeletal health.

In addition to those number one conservative treatment strategies, first-rate non-invasive techniques, on the facet of transcutaneous electric nerve stimulation (TENS), acupuncture, and rubdown treatment, additionally may be useful for managing neck pain. These complementary treatment alternatives can assist to relieve ache, promote rest, and aid the body's herbal restoration strategies. Integrating those remedy alternatives proper into a complete conservative treatment plan can assist to optimize effects and beautify the man or woman's normal nicely-being.

This chapter goals to provide a complete evaluation of these conservative treatment options, their underlying mechanisms, and the quality practices for using each approach. By information the severa conservative remedy techniques for neck ache, human beings and healthcare companies can paintings collectively to growth a customized remedy plan that addresses the specific wishes and dreams of the character, predominant to advanced function, reduced pain, and a higher awesome of lifestyles.

Over-the-counter (OTC) medicinal capsules are usually the number one line of remedy for slight to moderate neck pain. These medicinal capsules can assist reduce pain, irritation, and muscle anxiety via targeting amazing pathways worried in ache notion and infection. The maximum common OTC drug remedies for neck ache manage embody nonsteroidal anti inflammatory tablets (NSAIDs), acetaminophen, and topical analgesics.

NSAIDs, including ibuprofen and naproxen, work via blockading the manufacturing of prostaglandins, which might be materials that promote inflammation and boom ache sensitivity. These capsules inhibit the cyclooxygenase (COX) enzymes answerable for the synthesis of prostaglandins. NSAIDs are particularly effective in reducing infection, making them a certainly high-quality preference for neck pain due to conditions like muscle lines or cervical osteoarthritis.

Acetaminophen, moreover called paracetamol, is some other not unusual OTC ache reliever. While it is not as powerful at reducing contamination as NSAIDs, it is able to no matter the fact that offer relief from slight to mild pain. Acetaminophen works by using way of way of inhibiting the synthesis of prostaglandins inside the number one worried device, which in flip reduces the notion of pain. It may be used on my own or in aggregate with NSAIDs to provide extra entire pain treatment.

Topical analgesics, including lotions, gels, or patches, moreover may be used to manipulate neck pain. These merchandise frequently comprise active components like menthol, camphor, or capsaicin, which paintings thru stimulating nerve endings within the pores and skin, growing a sensation of warmth or coolness and short reducing ache belief. Some topical analgesics moreover consist of NSAIDs, that could offer localized anti-inflammatory effects.

It is vital to have a look at the endorsed dosages for the ones pills and to be privy to capability aspect consequences. For NSAIDs, not unusual component outcomes embody gastrointestinal troubles like heartburn, nausea, and belly ulcers. In a few cases, prolonged-time period use of NSAIDs also can result in kidney harm or stepped forward hazard of cardiovascular events. Acetaminophen, at the equal time as used inside encouraged dosages, generally has fewer facet consequences. However, immoderate use or combining it with alcohol can bring about liver toxicity.

To restriction the risk of component outcomes, it's far vital to apply OTC ache relievers best as directed and for the shortest period vital. Long-time period use need to be avoided except prescribed through a healthcare professional, who can display screen the man or woman's reaction to the medication and make certain that it is getting used competently and efficiently. In some times, a healthcare issuer may additionally moreover advise alternative or extra remedy alternatives to better cope with the underlying cause of the neck pain.

In instances in which over-the-counter (OTC) medicinal drugs do no longer offer enough consolation from neck ache, healthcare businesses can also moreover hold in thoughts prescribing stronger medicinal drugs. Prescription medicinal tablets for neck pain manage can embody prescription-strength nonsteroidal anti-inflammatory capsules (NSAIDs), muscle relaxants, and opioids, each with their specific mechanisms of movement and capacity facet results.

Prescription-power NSAIDs are much like their OTC opposite numbers but have a higher dosage, offering extra powerful anti inflammatory and pain-relieving results. Examples of prescription-power NSAIDs encompass diclofenac, ketorolac, and celecoxib. These capsules paintings via inhibiting the enzymes cyclooxygenase-1 (COX-1) and cyclooxygenase-2 (COX-2), which might be answerable for the producing of prostaglandins that promote infection and increase ache sensitivity. While those drug remedies may be more powerful in handling neck pain, moreover they carry a higher danger of side consequences, together with gastrointestinal bleeding, ulcers, and kidney damage. Therefore, prescription-energy NSAIDs should be used with warning and handiest underneath the supervision of a healthcare provider.

Muscle relaxants, which include cyclobenzaprine, tizanidine, and baclofen, are some unique elegance of prescription medicinal capsules that can be used for neck pain manage. These drug remedies paintings with the aid of using way of acting at the massive apprehensive machine to decrease

27

muscle tone and reduce muscle spasms, thereby providing comfort from neck ache because of muscle tension. Muscle relaxants can also assist improve the type of movement and everyday function of the neck. However, they might cause aspect results such as drowsiness, dizziness, and dry mouth. Patients taking muscle relaxants have to be monitored for the ones facet consequences, and dosage changes may be vital to lessen negative reactions.

Opioids, which incorporates oxycodone, hydrocodone, and morphine, are powerful pain relievers that can be prescribed for intense or continual neck ache that has now not spoke back to different remedies. Opioids art work with the resource of manner of binding to particular opioid receptors within the thoughts and spinal wire, inhibiting the transmission of ache indicators and offering ache remedy. They can be exceedingly effective in coping with excessive ache, however due to their capacity for addiction, abuse, and element effects, opioids should be prescribed with caution and simplest for quick-time period use.

Some commonplace component outcomes of opioids include drowsiness, dizziness, constipation, and respiration melancholy. Opioid-induced breathing despair may be existence-threatening, in particular in sufferers with pre-modern respiration situations or people who take one-of-a-kind drugs that could suppress breathing. Due to these risks, healthcare organizations want to cautiously reveal sufferers on opioid remedy and make suitable dosage adjustments to make certain affected person protection.

In a few instances, healthcare organizations may moreover prescribe awesome forms of medicinal drugs, including antidepressants or anticonvulsants, to control neck ache. These drugs, particularly tricyclic antidepressants and effective anticonvulsants like gabapentin and pregabalin, had been determined to be powerful in coping with neuropathic ache, which can be a detail of neck pain, specifically in instances of cervical radiculopathy. These medicinal tablets artwork with the useful resource of modulating ache signaling pathways in the nervous device, supplying ache relief without the risks related to opioids.

Prescription medicinal capsules can play an important position in handling neck ache even as OTC medicinal drugs are insufficient. These medicinal drugs embody prescription-energy NSAIDs, muscle relaxants, opioids, and, in a few times, antidepressants or anticonvulsants. Each beauty of medication has its specific mechanisms of movement, functionality factor outcomes, and problems for use. Healthcare agencies should cautiously have a look at the risks and benefits of each remedy, thinking of the individual affected person's dreams and medical information, to make certain stable and powerful neck It is vital for patients to comply with their healthcare issuer's guidelines regarding the prescribed remedy's dosage, frequency, and length of use. Open verbal exchange a few of the affected character and the healthcare issuer can help make certain that the selected remedy is efficiently managing neck pain on the identical time as minimizing component consequences. Regular observe-up appointments are crucial to reveal the affected character's development, compare the medicine's effectiveness, and make any vital modifications to the remedy plan.

In a few times, a aggregate of medicines can be prescribed to acquire most pleasurable ache remedy and deal with the best mechanisms contributing to neck pain. For instance, a affected person may be prescribed a muscle relaxant to reduce muscle spasms and an NSAID to cope with infection. It is important for patients to tell their healthcare companies of some different drugs they may be taking, which incorporates OTC medicinal pills and nutritional dietary supplements, to avoid capability drug interactions and negative consequences.

Prescription medicinal capsules should be used as part of a entire neck pain manage plan that could encompass bodily treatment, ergonomic modifications, and manner of existence changes. By combining these precise processes, patients can maximize their opportunities of undertaking ache comfort, restoring neck function, and stopping destiny episodes of neck pain.

Prescription drug treatments play a critical characteristic inside the manipulate of neck ache while conservative remedies, which incorporates OTC medicines, are inadequate. Through careful evaluation and tracking by way of healthcare groups, patients can use prescribed drugs efficiently and efficaciously to govern their neck pain. By incorporating those medicinal drugs proper into a complete treatment plan, sufferers can work inside the route of progressed neck feature, reduced ache, and an superior great of life.

Chapter 3: Physical Therapy And Rehabilitation

Techniques to Strengthen and Restore Neck Function

Physical treatment plays a crucial feature in handling neck pain and enhancing the first rate of life for affected people. Neck pain can arise from severa causes, such as muscle strain, bad posture, disc herniation, whiplash, and degenerative conditions along with osteoarthritis or spinal stenosis. As a non-invasive and holistic method, physical remedy goals to cope with the root motive of the ache and employs numerous techniques tailored to every affected person's precise needs.

The primary goals of bodily remedy for neck ache are to restore neck characteristic, lower pain, and save you destiny episodes of ache. To attain these desires, physical therapists make use of a combination of passive and energetic strategies that focus on the affected systems within the cervical backbone and surrounding gentle tissues. Passive techniques are the ones done thru manner of the therapist, which incorporates guide treatment or the usage of modalities, on the equal time as lively strategies require the affected individual's participation, which includes healing sporting activities.

Manual remedy techniques encompass masses of hands-on techniques, such as mild tissue mobilization, joint mobilization, and cervical traction. These strategies cause to relieve muscle tightness, improve joint mobility, and reduce stress on the cervical backbone, ultimately primary to reduced ache and multiplied feature. In conjunction with guide therapy, bodily therapists rent restoration sports designed to improve the affected person's kind of movement, make more potent supporting muscle tissues, and accurate postural imbalances that may be contributing to neck pain.

In addition to manual treatment and recovery wearing occasions, bodily therapists moreover utilize numerous modalities to control neck ache. These also can furthermore consist of warm temperature treatment, bloodless remedy, electric powered powered stimulation, and ultrasound remedy. Heat and bloodless remedy can help to loosen up muscle mass, increase blood go with the flow, reduce infection, and alleviate ache, on the identical time as electric powered powered stimulation and ultrasound treatment can provide greater ache remedy and sell tissue healing.

An crucial issue of bodily therapy for neck pain is the improvement of individualized remedy plans primarily based mostly on a complete assessment of the affected person's signs, manner of life, and scientific statistics. This customized technique guarantees that each affected individual receives the most suitable interventions for their specific desires and desires, maximizing the effectiveness of the treatment plan. Furthermore, physical therapists emphasize affected individual schooling and the improvement of domestic workout packages to empower patients to take an active characteristic in their restoration and save you future episodes of neck ache.

Physical treatment is a important thing of the whole treatment plan for people experiencing neck pain. By using a aggregate of manual treatment, recuperation carrying activities, and modalities, physical therapists can cope with the underlying reasons of neck ache, repair feature, and beautify the overall extraordinary of lifestyles for affected individuals. With a focal point on customized remedy plans and affected man or woman training, bodily remedy gives a holistic and non-invasive method to dealing with neck pain and stopping future episodes.

The preliminary assessment in bodily remedy is a crucial step in records the affected person's neck pain, because it permits the therapist to pick out out ability contributing elements and create a customized treatment plan. This entire evaluation tool includes numerous components, together with the collection of the affected individual's facts, a bodily exam, and, whilst essential, the usage of diagnostic imaging.

The series of the affected person's records is an vital detail of the initial evaluation. During this diploma, the bodily therapist will acquire records about the patient's signs and signs and symptoms, which include the onset, period, frequency, and intensity of the ache. This can also additionally moreover contain using ache scales or questionnaires to quantify the affected character's pain levels. The therapist will even inquire approximately any preceding episodes of neck pain, beyond remedies, and their effects.

The affected man or woman's way of lifestyles and occupational factors also are applicable, as the ones can significantly impact neck pain. For example, a sedentary lifestyle or a task that calls for prolonged sitting or repetitive neck movements can make a contribution to the improvement or exacerbation of neck pain. The therapist will do not forget those factors while designing the remedy plan, as addressing those way of life and occupational factors can be essential for prolonged-time period pain alleviation and prevention.

The medical information of the affected man or woman is some specific crucial issue of the preliminary assessment. The therapist will ask approximately any pre-present scientific situations, preceding surgical processes or accidents, and the affected individual's modern treatment regimen. This records permits the therapist to apprehend capability contraindications to specific remedy techniques and to do not forget any comorbidities which can have an impact at the affected person's neck ache or remedy results.

The physical examination is the subsequent factor of the initial evaluation. During this examination, the bodily therapist will verify the affected man or woman's type of motion inside the cervical backbone, collectively with flexion, extension, lateral flexion, and rotation. The therapist might also even examine the energy of the neck and better decrease again muscle businesses, as vulnerable point in the ones muscle corporations can contribute to pain and disease. Postural evaluation is each different crucial element of the physical examination, as bad posture can region excessive pressure at the cervical backbone and surrounding mild tissues.

Palpation of the cervical backbone and surrounding gentle tissues is an essential technique used by the bodily therapist all through the initial evaluation. By manually inspecting the affected individual's neck, the therapist can choose out regions of tenderness, muscle spasm, or joint regulations that can be contributing to the affected individual's neck pain.

In some instances, the physical therapist can also request diagnostic imaging, which include X-rays, MRI, or CT scans, to gather a clearer knowledge of the underlying motive of the affected individual's neck ache. These imaging studies can help to pick out out out unique structural problems, which incorporates disc herniations, bone spurs, or spinal stenosis, that may be contributing to the affected character's symptoms and signs and symptoms. The therapist will use this records to manual the treatment plan and make certain that the most suitable interventions are employed.

Overall, the preliminary assessment is an entire machine that allows the bodily therapist to gain an extensive information of the affected man or woman's neck ache and its functionality contributing factors. This facts is treasured in growing a custom designed remedy plan that addresses the affected person's unique goals and optimizes their rehabilitation effects.

Establishing sensible and feasible goals for rehabilitation is a critical element of the physical treatment method. By running together with the affected individual, the bodily therapist can better apprehend the patient's priorities, expectancies, and boundaries, that allows you to inform the improvement of an individualized remedy plan.

During the reason-setting approach, the therapist and affected individual will talk each short-time period and prolonged-time period objectives. Short-time period desires might also moreover attention on immediately pain comfort, enhancing form of motion, and lowering muscle stiffness or spasms. Long-time period desires, but, regularly include restoring full neck function, improving energy and flexibility, enhancing posture, and stopping destiny episodes of neck pain.

The therapist will remember severa elements at the same time as putting those desires, together with the affected person's age, modern health, profession, and each day sports activities sports. For example, an workplace worker who spends prolonged hours within the the front of a pc may additionally require particular ergonomic modifications and posture correction wearing occasions, at the same time as an athlete may also moreover want game-precise rehabilitation to go returned to their pre-harm degree of common universal overall performance.

Once dreams had been established, the therapist will layout a customized treatment plan tailored to the affected man or woman's specific desires. This plan will consist of a mixture of evidence-based totally completely strategies, including guide remedy, restoration physical video games, and adjunctive treatment plans, to optimize neck characteristic, alleviate pain, and save you recurrence.

The remedy plan will begin with a focal point on ache comfort and manipulate, which also can incorporate the use of modalities like warmness, bloodless, or electric stimulation, further to slight guide remedy strategies. As the affected individual's pain subsides and their tolerance for movement will boom, the therapist will steadily introduce healing sports activities sports to decorate style of movement, flexibility, and power. The choice of wearing activities can be based totally at the patient's unique deficits and beneficial barriers, as diagnosed at some stage in the preliminary assessment.

In addition to addressing the bodily factors of neck ache, the therapist might also recall the affected individual's psychosocial factors, together with pressure, tension, and melancholy, which also can make a contribution to or exacerbate their signs. The remedy plan may additionally additionally include strategies for stress manipulate, rest techniques, and coping abilties to help the affected individual manage these factors greater efficiently.

Throughout the route of remedy, the physical therapist will continuously screen and reconsider the affected character's progress, making changes to the remedy plan as preferred. This ongoing evaluation guarantees that the affected person's desires remain sensible and ability, and that the remedy plan stays effective in addressing their unique needs. Regular verbal exchange a few of the affected character and the therapist is essential to facilitate this method and make certain that the patient remains engaged and committed to their rehabilitation journey.

Soft tissue mobilization (STM) is a essential manual remedy approach utilized by physical therapists to address neck ache and disease. STM focuses on manipulating the muscles, ligaments, and fascia in the cervical area, that might assist alleviate discomfort, decorate mobility, and beautify the overall function of the neck. This hands-on method employs a number of techniques, which encompass mild pressure, rhythmic stretching, and sustained holds, to aim mild tissues that may be contributing to neck pain.

The number one desires of slight tissue mobilization are to launch tightness, alleviate muscle spasms, and sell blood go along with the drift to the affected location. By utilising focused strain to unique areas of anxiety, the therapist can encourage the relaxation of shrunk muscular tissues and boom the extensibility of the surrounding connective tissue. This can bring about advanced muscle balance and decreased stress on the cervical spine. Additionally, selling blood go with the flow to the region allows deliver critical nutrients and oxygen, which can manual the recovery way and decrease inflammation.

Soft tissue mobilization also can help to interrupt up scar tissue and adhesions that may be contributing to neck ache. Scar tissue and adhesions are the body's natural reaction to harm and might shape due to trauma, surgical treatment, or continual irritation. While the ones formations help to stabilize and guard the injured area, they can also bring about limited motion, reduced tissue flexibility, and superior ache. By using specialised STM techniques, which consist of go with the flow-friction rubdown and myofascial launch, the therapist can gently smash down those restrictive systems and restore normal tissue mobility.

It is vital to phrase that the effectiveness of mild tissue mobilization relies upon at the talent and records of the therapist, similarly to the affected person's character goals and tolerance. To gain gold popular effects, the therapist need to use appropriate strategies and pressure, tailor-made to the affected man or woman's consolation degree and unique situation. Furthermore, ongoing verbal exchange a number of the therapist and the patient is critical to make certain that the treatment remains effective and comfortable inside the route of the technique.

Chapter 4: Alternative And Complementary Therapies

Acupuncture, Massage, and Chiropractic Care for Neck Pain Relief

Neck ache is a enormous musculoskeletal illness that influences a large a part of the populace. Various factors can make a contribution to neck pain, in conjunction with muscle traces, degenerative disc ailment, herniated discs, and spinal stenosis. Conventional scientific remedies like remedy and bodily treatment are frequently the first line of safety for handling neck pain. However, possibility and complementary treatments can also play a important feature in addressing this circumstance. These treatment options, which include acupuncture, rubdown, and chiropractic care, have increasingly more received interest because of their ability blessings in ache consolation and everyday well-being. This bankruptcy goals to offer a complete examine of these remedies and the current medical proof helping their efficacy in treating neck pain.

Alternative and complementary remedies encompass a numerous kind of treatment modalities that are not commonly considered a part of conventional remedy. They are frequently used together with well-known scientific treatments to enhance their effectiveness, deal with capacity factor consequences, and enhance the general pleasant of lifestyles for sufferers. In the context of neck ache, opportunity and complementary remedy plans can help lessen ache depth, decorate useful mobility, and sell a sense of relaxation and strain comfort. These benefits can be mainly precious for human beings with chronic neck ache, who frequently enjoy a complicated interplay of bodily, intellectual, and social factors that contribute to their state of affairs.

The developing interest in opportunity and complementary restoration strategies for neck ache may be attributed to numerous factors. First, there is growing public attention and make contact with for for non-pharmacological and non-invasive treatment alternatives, specially in moderate of the opioid catastrophe and issues about the lengthy-time period safety and efficacy of positive medicinal pills. Second, a growing body of medical studies has started to provide an explanation for the mechanisms and medical benefits of these remedies, lending credibility to their use in scientific exercising. Third, many healthcare carriers and sufferers are embracing a extra holistic and patient-centered technique to care, which acknowledges the importance of addressing the entire man or woman, together with their bodily, emotional, and social well-being.

Despite the capability advantages of possibility and complementary remedies for neck ache, their use in medical exercise is not without stressful situations. One widespread venture is the variety within the quality and rigor of studies research, that may make it hard to draw definitive conclusions about the efficacy and protection of wonderful restoration methods. Additionally, there is mostly a lack of standardized remedy protocols and hints, making it tough for healthcare groups to decide the maximum appropriate remedy path for his or her sufferers. Finally, get admission to to possibility and complementary treatments can be restrained via manner of factors together with insurance insurance, enterprise availability, and affected person data and alternatives.

In slight of these stressful situations, it is essential to seriously appraise the available medical evidence for opportunity and complementary remedy options for neck ache and to have interaction in a collaborative and knowledgeable choice-making device with patients. This economic ruin will delve deeper into 3 appreciably used treatments – acupuncture, rubdown, and chiropractic care – analyzing their theoretical foundations, clinical evidence, and sensible troubles for neck pain remedy. By statistics the modern-day country of expertise and last open to new research and views, healthcare providers can higher assist their sufferers in navigating the complicated panorama of neck ache control and reaching nice effects.

Acupuncture is a traditional Chinese treatment workout that has been used for lots of years to deal with severa health situations, collectively with neck pain. It includes the insertion of skinny needles into precise elements on the frame, known as acupuncture points or acupoints. The underlying principle of acupuncture is based absolutely at the concept of Qi (recommended "chee"), this is considered critical power or existence force that flows through channels, or meridians, in the frame. These meridians shape a complicated community that connects numerous organs and frame components. When Qi is blocked or disrupted, it can result in ache, infection, or disease. Acupuncture desires to repair the stability and go with the flow of Qi via stimulating acupoints, as a result promoting recuperation and ache consolation.

Recent research has supplied insights into the viable mechanisms thru which acupuncture may additionally provide ache consolation. One of the number one mechanisms is the discharge of endogenous opioids, which is probably the frame's herbal painkillers. When acupuncture needles are inserted into acupoints, they stimulate the discharge of endorphins, enkephalins, and dynorphins, which can be endogenous opioid peptides. These substances bind to opioid receptors within the demanding tool and correctly lessen the belief of ache.

Another proposed mechanism of acupuncture's pain-relieving effect is the modulation of the pain signaling pathway. Pain signs and symptoms are transmitted from the internet site of harm or inflammation to the mind through a chain of nerve fibers and synapses. Acupuncture is idea to regulate the ache transmission technique through inhibiting the activation of certain pain pathways or with the aid of stimulating the release of neurotransmitters, which include serotonin and norepinephrine, which have analgesic effects.

Additionally, acupuncture has been proven to beautify nearby blood go with the flow, that may help sell healing and reduce infection on the website online of ache. By developing blood flow, acupuncture can deliver oxygen and nutrients to the affected location greater efficaciously and facilitate the removal of waste products and inflammatory mediators, which may additionally moreover contribute to the bargain of ache and soreness.

Furthermore, acupuncture has been placed to have anti-inflammatory results, which can also play a feature in its potential to alleviate neck ache. It is normally recommended that acupuncture can modulate the discharge of seasoned-inflammatory cytokines, consisting of tumor necrosis component-alpha (TNF-α) and interleukin-6 (IL-6), which can be worried within the inflammatory reaction. By reducing the levels of these seasoned-inflammatory cytokines, acupuncture can also help to reduce infection and, consequently, alleviate ache.

It should be cited that the suitable mechanisms via which acupuncture relieves neck ache are even though now not without a doubt understood, and extra studies is needed to make clear the best pathways and techniques concerned. Nonetheless, the modern-day proof indicates that acupuncture can provide ache comfort via a combination of neurochemical, neurophysiological, and circulatory mechanisms, making it a possibly precious remedy desire for those affected by neck pain.

The effectiveness of acupuncture in treating neck ache has been a topic of hobby in numerous scientific trials and systematic opinions. A exquisite systematic evaluate and meta-analysis published in 2017 analyzed information from 22 randomized managed trials (RCTs) to assess the efficacy of acupuncture for neck ache. This entire evaluation positioned that acupuncture outperformed sham acupuncture, inactive treatment, and geared up list manage in reducing neck pain intensity and enhancing characteristic. The researchers concluded that acupuncture can be considered a possible treatment preference for neck ache remedy.

Another systematic review, posted in 2020, in addition investigated the effectiveness of acupuncture in treating neck pain. This evaluation protected 27 RCTs and in addition concluded that acupuncture have become effective in assuaging neck pain and enhancing neck function, with a specific emphasis on its benefits for patients with persistent neck pain. This compare moreover highlighted that acupuncture may additionally want to potentially reduce the want for ache medications and improve the general best of life for sufferers suffering from neck ache.

Chapter 5: Cervical Traction And Orthotic Devices

The Role of Supportive Aids in Neck Pain Treatment

Cervical traction and orthotic gadgets have acquired prominence in brand new years due to their potential to alleviate neck ache and pain, sell recovery, and restore the everyday functioning of the cervical backbone. These supportive aids are an imperative part of a whole treatment plan that normally includes one-of-a-type conservative interventions which incorporates treatment control, physical remedy, and way of life changes.

Cervical traction is a therapeutic technique that objectives to decompress the cervical spine through lightly stretching the neck muscle corporations and ligaments. This approach helps reduce strain on the nerves, alleviate pain, beautify blood waft, and facilitate the recuperation of injured tissues. Cervical traction may be achieved the use of mechanical gadgets or manual strategies, depending at the affected individual's needs and the healthcare expert's tips.

Orthotic devices, commonly called cervical collars or neck braces, are designed to provide help and balance to the neck through proscribing motion and keeping proper alignment. These gadgets can be employed for various functions, which incorporates immobilization following trauma or surgical treatment, offering temporary comfort from ache for the duration of each day sports, and preserving alignment inside the course of the recovery method.

Both cervical traction and orthotic gadgets have their signs, contraindications, and precautions that healthcare experts need to bear in mind to make sure affected individual protection and treatment efficacy. The desire of intervention and the right form of traction or orthotic device used want to be primarily based at the affected man or woman's person condition, signs and signs and symptoms, and treatment goals. It is important to tailor the treatment plan to the affected man or woman's particular wishes and display their improvement at a few stage in the path of remedy.

The proof supporting using cervical traction and orthotic devices in neck ache control remains evolving. While some studies have installed promising consequences, in particular for quick-time period ache treatment and advanced characteristic, the lengthy-term benefits of these interventions have now not been well-hooked up. More high-quality research is needed to affirm the efficacy of cervical traction and orthotic devices and to pick out out the only treatment protocols and gadgets for precise neck ache conditions.

In this financial ruin, we're capable of find out the requirements of cervical traction and severa orthotic gadgets in greater element, communicate their warning signs, contraindications, and precautions, and feature a take a look at the cutting-edge-day evidence helping their use in neck pain remedy. We can even highlight the importance of a whole, multimodal approach to neck ache control that consists of cervical traction and orthotic devices as part of a broader treatment plan.

Cervical traction is a non-invasive therapy that has been used for decades to assist alleviate neck ache via targeted on the cervical spine's underlying systems. The vital principles of cervical traction encompass lightly stretching the cervical backbone, decompressing the intervertebral discs, and decreasing strain on the nerves. This stretching and decompression can offer remedy from pain, beautify blood move, and sell the restoration of injured tissues. There are primary forms of cervical traction: mechanical and manual.

Mechanical cervical traction is run the usage of gadgets that exercise a managed pressure to stretch the neck muscle agencies and ligaments. This shape of traction can be non-stop or intermittent, relying on the affected character's wishes and comfort diploma. Mechanical traction gadgets may be further divided into over-the-door and supine traction gadgets. Over-the-door traction gadgets are transportable devices designed for home use, in which the affected character wears a head halter linked to a pulley tool set up on a door. The traction pressure is generated through such as weights to the device, and the remedy duration and frequency may be custom designed in step with the clinician's tips. On the opposite hand, supine traction gadgets allow sufferers to lie down within the direction of remedy, making sure a greater comfortable and managed enjoy. These devices regularly function integrated controls that permit the patient or the therapist to adjust the traction pressure and duration. Supine traction gadgets may be applied in medical settings or at home, with a few models designed for transportable use.

Manual cervical traction is completed thru a expert healthcare professional, along with a bodily therapist or chiropractor, who makes use of their fingers to use a controlled stress to the affected person's neck. The therapist adjusts the traction stress, direction, and length based totally on the affected person's signs and symptoms and reaction to treatment. Manual cervical traction lets in for more customization of the remedy but calls for normal visits to a healthcare professional.

One of the primary benefits of cervical traction is that it is able to be tailored to the precise goals of each affected character. Factors along with the affected man or woman's age, traditional health, and the severity of their neck pain can affect the shape of cervical traction hired, further to the frequency and duration of treatment classes. Furthermore, cervical traction may be blended with exclusive remedies, which incorporates physical remedy, remedy, and complementary treatment options, to create a entire and individualized remedy plan.

The effectiveness of cervical traction is supported through diverse clinical studies.

Research has verified that it can offer brief-term pain relief and advanced function for patients with conditions which includes cervical radiculopathy and herniated discs. However, more first rate research is needed to verify its prolonged-time period efficacy and establish maximum fine remedy protocols.

Cervical traction is a non-invasive remedy that gives a viable preference for patients tormented by neck pain. By lightly stretching the cervical spine and decompressing the intervertebral discs, cervical traction can relieve pain, beautify blood glide, and sell the healing of injured tissues. The desire between mechanical and manual cervical traction is primarily based upon at the patient's wishes, opportunities, and the supply of informed healthcare professionals.

Mechanical cervical traction is a healing method that employs specifically designed devices to use managed pressure to the cervical spine, grade by grade stretching the neck muscle tissue and ligaments. This method of traction helps alleviate neck pain through decompressing the intervertebral discs, decreasing pressure at the nerves, and selling relaxation of the muscles. Mechanical cervical traction gadgets provide the gain of being more precise and consistent in evaluation to guide traction, as they allow for better manipulate over the pressure, period, and frequency of the completed traction.

Mechanical cervical traction can be applied both constantly or intermittently, counting on the affected person's desires and restoration dreams. Continuous traction involves the use of a ordinary pressure to the cervical backbone for an prolonged length, on the identical time as intermittent traction applies the pressure in cycles, with durations of traction observed thru intervals of rest. The depth of the traction strain may be adjusted consistent with the affected individual's consolation diploma and the particular remedy desires.

Mechanical traction gadgets may be significantly classified into classes: over-the-door and supine traction gadgets. Over-the-door traction gadgets are easy, portable devices that can be with out hassle set up at home. They encompass a head halter that suits for the duration of the affected man or woman's head and a pulley system mounted on a door. The traction strain is generated thru together with weights to the pulley machine, and the pressure may be adjusted with the resource of converting the quantity of weight used. Over-the-door traction gadgets are pretty much less high-priced and convenient for domestic use however won't provide the equal degree of control and precision as supine traction devices.

Supine traction devices, alternatively, are extra superior gadgets that allow patients to lie down in a few unspecified time within the destiny of the traction treatment, ensuring a extra snug and managed enjoy. These gadgets regularly include integrated virtual controls that allow the affected person or the therapist to alter the traction strain, length, and cycle settings. Some supine traction devices moreover have extra abilities, collectively with heating elements, vibration, or infrared treatment, to decorate the therapeutic effects of the treatment.

Supine traction devices can be utilized in clinical settings, along with bodily therapy clinics or hospitals, similarly to at domestic, with a few fashions in particular designed for portable use. While supine traction gadgets have a propensity to be more luxurious than over-the-door devices, they offer a higher stage of precision, control, and comfort, making them a well-known desire for each healthcare professionals and sufferers.

Mechanical cervical traction gadgets offer a non-invasive and controlled approach to assuaging neck ache thru utilizing particular, adjustable force to the cervical spine. Both over-the-door and supine traction gadgets have their benefits and limitations, and the choice among them relies upon on elements inclusive of affected man or woman consolation, recuperation dreams, and rate range. As part of a complete neck ache remedy plan, mechanical cervical traction can complement great interventions, which includes bodily treatment, treatment, and way of existence adjustments, to sell restoration and repair everyday characteristic.

Over-the-door traction devices have turn out to be well-known for domestic use, as they provide an available and cost-effective solution for patients trying to find treatment from neck pain. These transportable devices include a head halter, a pulley device, and a hard and fast of weights. The head halter is designed to cradle the affected individual's head securely, meting out the traction pressure calmly throughout the neck. The pulley gadget, that is installed on a door, is liable for translating the load-delivered about stress into vertical traction at the cervical backbone.

To use an over-the-door traction unit, the affected individual should first communicate over with a healthcare professional to determine the perfect traction pressure, treatment duration, and frequency. This statistics is vital for customizing the treatment plan and making sure that the affected man or woman opinions high-quality advantages from the treatment at the same time as minimizing the hazard of damage.

Once the affected individual has obtained their clinician's recommendations, they are able to set up the over-the-door traction unit at domestic by way of manner of following the manufacturer's instructions. It is critical to ensure that the door is strong and securely closed to save you accidents for the duration of treatment. The affected individual have to then cautiously regulate the top halter to fit effects and securely round their head, averting any pointless stress at the jaw or face. The chin strap must be cushty however no longer overly tight to allow for herbal jaw motion and swallowing.

After adjusting the pinnacle halter, the affected man or woman can join the pulley gadget to the door and be a part of the top halter to the pulley using the provided straps or hooks. The clinician-recommended weights can then be brought to the traction system, so as to create a vertical stress that gently stretches the neck muscle businesses and ligaments. It is essential to start with a lower traction strain and grade by grade increase it over the years, as tolerated.

During the treatment, the patient should be seated resultseasily with their lower lower back supported and their toes flat at the floor. They ought to keep a comfortable posture, with their head and neck aligned with the spine. The period of every remedy session can range relying at the healthcare expert's pointers, however commonly, intervals ultimate among 15 and 1/2-hour. The affected person need to reveal their symptoms and symptoms and signs and symptoms and speak any discomfort or detrimental results to their healthcare employer.

The effectiveness of over-the-door traction gadgets for neck ache comfort may additionally range depending at the man or woman affected character's state of affairs and the underlying motive of their pain. Some patients also can enjoy big comfort from their signs and symptoms and signs and symptoms, whilst others can also additionally require more interventions together with bodily remedy, remedy, or alternative remedies. As with any remedy, it's miles vital for the affected man or woman to examine their healthcare expert's hints and adhere to the prescribed remedy plan to acquire the best effects.

Supine traction gadgets are designed to offer a more comfortable and controlled revel in for patients, as they permit them to lie down in some unspecified time in the future of remedy. This position has severa advantages over the sitting or repute positions applied in different traction techniques, which include over-the-door traction gadgets. In the supine feature, the affected character's backbone is in a extra impartial alignment, which allows to distribute the traction strain greater lightly at some stage in the cervical backbone. Additionally, this position lets in for higher relaxation of the neck muscular tissues, which can decorate the effectiveness of the traction treatment.

These supine traction gadgets often come prepared with integrated controls that permit the affected man or woman or the therapist to alter the traction pressure and duration precisely. This customization is essential to offer the simplest treatment while minimizing the chance of harm or pain. The traction pressure can be step by step advanced over time because the affected man or woman's tolerance improves, and the duration of every session can be adjusted in keeping with the clinician's pointers.

Supine traction gadgets are bendy and may be utilized in severa settings, which include medical environments and at home. In scientific settings, which incorporates physical treatment clinics or rehabilitation centers, the therapist can carefully reveal the affected man or woman's development and make critical adjustments to the traction parameters. They can also offer hands-on help and steerage to make certain right positioning and approach.

For home use, a few supine traction unit fashions are designed for portability, making them easy to installation and keep. These domestic-based totally absolutely gadgets regularly encompass sure commands for safe and powerful use. However, sufferers want to are in search of recommendation from their healthcare business enterprise earlier than beginning a home traction application to make sure they get keep of suitable steering at the right technique and remedy parameters.

In addition to the adjustable traction stress and length, a few supine traction devices offer superior competencies, which incorporates the capacity to exchange the attitude of traction. This functionality can target particular areas of the cervical backbone more successfully and permits for the remedy of numerous neck ache situations. Another function determined in some gadgets is the usage of pneumatic or virtual structures to manipulate the traction pressure. These structures can offer more precise control over the traction parameters and can provide a smoother, extra comfortable enjoy for the affected person.

Despite the severa benefits of supine traction gadgets, it's miles vital to apprehend that they'll not be appropriate for all patients or neck pain conditions. Certain contraindications and precautions, as stated earlier on this financial disaster, ought to be considered before the usage of any cervical traction remedy. Patients ought to art work intently with their healthcare provider to determine if supine traction is appropriate for his or her specific state of affairs and to increase a custom designed remedy plan tailor-made to their individual desires.

Manual cervical traction is a healing approach finished thru way of educated healthcare specialists, which encompass bodily therapists, chiropractors, or osteopathic physicians. This palms-on technique consists of the software of a managed force to the affected person's neck to gently stretch the cervical spine, decompress the intervertebral discs, and alleviate pressure on the nerves. This method targets to lessen ache, improve mobility, and enhance the restoration technique in sufferers with neck pain.

During a guide cervical traction session, the healthcare expert positions the affected man or woman clearly, each seated or lying down, depending at the practitioner's choice and the affected individual's consolation. The therapist then makes use of their fingers to stabilize the affected man or woman's head at the same time as the usage of a controlled stress to the neck. The traction stress may be directed longitudinally (along the period of the backbone), laterally (in the direction of the rims), or at a particular attitude primarily based totally on the affected man or woman's signs and symptoms and symptoms and symptoms and anatomical problems.

One of the advantages of guide cervical traction is the capability to personalize the treatment steady with the affected person's desires. The therapist can modify the traction stress, route, and duration primarily based on the affected character's signs and symptoms, response to remedy, and regular consolation. Additionally, the therapist can display display the affected person's improvement within the route of the remedy, taking into consideration real-time modifications and modifications as wanted.

Manual cervical traction also lets in the healthcare expert to consist of various remedy modalities into the consultation, which includes smooth tissue mobilization, joint mobilization, or restoration wearing sports. This protected technique permits for a more whole remedy plan, focused on a couple of factors of the affected man or woman's neck ache and disorder.

Despite the advantages of guide cervical traction, there are some boundaries to don't forget. One of the primary drawbacks is the requirement for normal visits to a healthcare expert, which can be hard for patients with confined get right of access to to care or busy schedules. Additionally, the effectiveness of manual cervical traction may be inspired via the practitioner's ability and revel in, probably predominant to variable consequences.

As with any recovery intervention, the fulfillment of manual cervical traction is primarily based upon on proper affected individual choice and adherence to treatment guidelines. Healthcare experts have to don't forget the affected person's particular situation, any contraindications to traction, and the affected man or woman's normal goals and alternatives while identifying the most suitable treatment plan.

Manual cervical traction is a treasured remedy choice for patients with neck ache, presenting a customized, palms-on technique to care. Although it requires regular visits to a healthcare professional, the advantages of this technique, specially whilst mixed with one of a kind healing interventions, can bring about large upgrades in ache, mobility, and elegant splendid of life for plenty patients.

Cervical traction is a valuable healing preference for patients experiencing diverse neck ache situations. One such situation is cervical radiculopathy, which arises even as nerve roots in the cervical spine emerge as compressed or irritated. Cervical traction can alleviate the stress on the nerve roots, thereby presenting remedy from pain, numbness, and weak point radiating to the arms or hands.

Another indication for cervical traction is cervical spondylosis, a degenerative situation characterized by the wear and tear of spinal discs and aspect joints within the neck. Cervical traction can assist lessen joint stiffness, decompress the affected spinal segments, and enhance neck mobility in patients with spondylosis. Similarly, traction can be useful for sufferers with herniated or bulging cervical discs, as it could create space between the vertebrae and alleviate strain at the affected discs.

Cervical traction also can be useful for people with factor joint syndrome, a circumstance related to infection and ache within the facet joints of the cervical spine. By gently stretching the neck muscle organizations and ligaments, traction can reduce muscle spasms, alleviate joint pain, and promote a more balanced alignment of the cervical backbone. Patients with muscle spasms or traces and whiplash-related troubles also can gain from cervical traction, as it is able to help relieve ache and beautify range of motion.

Despite the recuperation benefits of cervical traction for various neck ache situations, it is essential to don't forget contraindications and precautions earlier than beginning remedy. Cervical traction need for use with warning or avoided in times of acute neck trauma or instability, as it can exacerbate the harm or compromise the structural integrity of the cervical spine.

Similarly, patients with rheumatoid arthritis or different inflammatory situations affecting the cervical spine have to workout caution even as thinking about cervical traction. Traction may additionally additionally likely get worse infection, leading to accelerated pain and joint harm. Additionally, individuals with cervical backbone malignancies or infections should avoid cervical traction, as it can make contributions to the unfold of cancer cells or infectious sellers.

Vertebral artery insufficiency, a situation characterised with the aid of decreased blood waft to the mind due to narrowing or occlusion of the vertebral arteries, is a few specific contraindication for cervical traction. Traction can exacerbate this example through further reducing blood drift, thereby growing the danger of stroke or unique neurological complications.

Chapter 6: Medication Management

Analgesics, Anti-Inflammatories, and Muscle Relaxants

Neck pain is a desired problem that influences tens of millions of human beings international, appreciably impacting their nice of lifestyles and each day functioning. Various factors can make a contribution to neck ache, together with horrific posture, muscle strain, degenerative situations, nerve compression, and accidents. Medication manipulate is a cornerstone of treatment for neck pain, often employed in mixture with other conservative treatment alternatives collectively with bodily therapy, lifestyle changes, and complementary and opportunity medication.

The primary goals of medication manage for neck ache include ache comfort, bargain of contamination, and facilitation of muscle rest. To benefit these desires, healthcare companies ought to don't forget the underlying motive of the neck ache, the severity and duration of symptoms and signs, and any applicable affected individual factors which includes age, clinical facts, and functionality contraindications. By tailoring medicine regimens to the individual patient, healthcare vendors can optimize ache comfort and purposeful improvement even as minimizing the threat of factor outcomes and headaches.

Medication manage for neck pain includes a good sized kind of pharmaceutical shops, every with its unique mechanisms of motion, signs and symptoms, and capability factor outcomes. Some common medicinal drug lessons used in the control of neck ache embody analgesics, nonsteroidal anti inflammatory capsules (NSAIDs), corticosteroids, muscle relaxants, antidepressants, and anticonvulsants. These medicines can be used on my own or in combination, relying on the particular goals of the affected individual and the individual of their neck pain.

In addition to statistics the numerous kinds of medicinal capsules to be had for neck pain manage, healthcare groups and patients have to moreover be privy to the functionality element effects and interactions associated with those capsules. This knowledge lets in knowledgeable choice-making and ensures the secure and powerful use of medication. Furthermore, it's miles crucial to recognize that treatment manipulate is regularly absolutely one detail of a complete remedy plan for neck pain. Integrating medicinal drugs with extraordinary conservative restoration strategies, which include bodily treatment, exercising, and posture exchange, can help patients benefit final pain consolation and lengthy-term beneficial improvement.

Medication control is an essential component of neck ache remedy, encompassing a severa array of pharmaceutical dealers designed to alleviate pain, lessen irritation, and sell muscle relaxation. By know-how the numerous drug treatments to be had, their mechanisms of motion, and functionality thing effects, healthcare corporations and sufferers can art work collectively to increase strong and effective remedy plans tailored to the man or woman's unique desires. Combining treatment manipulate with other conservative treatments can help sufferers gather the terrific possible results in their journey toward advanced neck health and decreased pain.

Acetaminophen, moreover referred to as paracetamol, is a widely used over-the-counter (OTC) analgesic and antipyretic medicine. As one of the maximum not unusual pain-consolation medicinal pills, it's far frequently the number one line of remedy for mild to slight neck ache. The tremendous use of acetaminophen can be attributed to its protection profile, ease of get right of entry to, and low price.

The unique mechanism of motion of acetaminophen remains unclear. However, it's far believed to include the inhibition of prostaglandin synthesis in the maximum crucial worried device. Prostaglandins are lipid compounds that play a important characteristic in contamination and pain notion. They are responsible for sensitizing ache receptors, and inhibiting their synthesis can successfully lessen pain perception. This inhibition is idea to upward thrust up commonly within the important concerned gadget, with minimal effect on peripheral prostaglandin production, which distinguishes acetaminophen from nonsteroidal anti inflammatory pills (NSAIDs).

Acetaminophen is usually taken into consideration constant whilst used as directed, with a low prevalence of element results. The most not unusual aspect effects are generally moderate and encompass nausea and headache. However, lengthy-term use or immoderate doses can result in hepatotoxicity (liver damage) and, in uncommon times, acute liver failure. This chance is specially concerning while each day doses exceed 4,000 milligrams (mg) for adults or on the equal time as acetaminophen is blended with special medicines that also incorporate acetaminophen, which includes cold and flu remedies. To lessen the risk of liver damage, it's far critical for sufferers to comply with the advocated dosing pointers and be cautious whilst the use of more than one medicinal tablets containing acetaminophen.

Furthermore, people with pre-present liver ailment, chronic alcohol intake, or who're the usage of medication that bring about liver enzymes, including a few anticonvulsants and tuberculosis pills, may be at a better hazard of growing hepatotoxicity with acetaminophen use. In those times, a decrease maximum each day dose may be encouraged, and close monitoring of liver feature is critical.

Patients want to moreover be aware of the functionality for drug interactions with acetaminophen. For example, the blood-thinning impact of warfarin, an anticoagulant medicine, may be more appropriate by way of using the concurrent use of acetaminophen. As a end result, it is vital for human beings taking warfarin or similar medicinal capsules to speak over with their healthcare employer earlier than the usage of acetaminophen.

Acetaminophen is a substantially used analgesic which can provide powerful comfort for mild to mild neck ache. However, it's far crucial for sufferers to paste to the advocated dosing pointers and be vigilant for capability drug interactions and the chance of hepatotoxicity. As with any remedy, it's miles important to go to a healthcare expert before starting, stopping, or converting any treatment regular for neck pain.

Nonsteroidal anti-inflammatory capsules (NSAIDs) are a widely applied elegance of drug treatments that provide each analgesic and anti-inflammatory consequences, making them in particular beneficial for addressing neck ache. NSAIDs paintings thru inhibiting the activity of cyclooxygenase (COX) enzymes, which play a vital function within the manufacturing of prostaglandins. Prostaglandins are lipid compounds that make a contribution to irritation and ache. By inhibiting COX enzymes, NSAIDs reduce prostaglandin synthesis, main to a decrease in irritation and ache.

There are important varieties of COX enzymes: COX-1 and COX-2. COX-1 is accountable for the producing of prostaglandins that protect the belly lining and assist blood clotting, while COX-2 is accountable for generating prostaglandins that motive contamination and ache. Traditional NSAIDs, which incorporates ibuprofen, naproxen, and aspirin, inhibit every COX-1 and COX-2 enzymes, presenting ache remedy and anti inflammatory effects.

Selective COX-2 inhibitors, which incorporates celecoxib, particularly intention the COX-2 enzyme, ensuing in a reduction of irritation and ache with out impacting the protective abilties of COX-1. This selectivity can also additionally bring about fewer gastrointestinal issue results as compared to conventional NSAIDs. However, selective COX-2 inhibitors have been associated with an advanced hazard of cardiovascular activities, necessitating cautious interest of affected person chance factors at the same time as prescribing the ones medicinal drugs.

NSAIDs can be powerful for short-time period remedy of acute neck ache, mainly while inflammation is gift. They may be used for numerous reasons of neck pain, which incorporates muscle strains, ligament sprains, and degenerative situations together with osteoarthritis. Over-the-counter NSAIDs are generally the number one line of treatment, whilst prescription-energy NSAIDs may be taken into consideration for added excessive or chronic ache.

While NSAIDs can offer exceptional remedy for neck pain sufferers, their lengthy-term use carries capability dangers. One of the primary issues with extended NSAID use is the prolonged hazard of gastrointestinal (GI) complications. These headaches can variety from moderate gastritis to greater immoderate issues together with peptic ulcers and GI bleeding. This danger is in particular heightened in aged patients, humans with a information of GI problems, and people taking concomitant drugs that would worsen the stomach lining, together with corticosteroids or anticoagulants.

In addition to GI complications, prolonged-term use of NSAIDs has been associated with other capability side results, which includes renal impairment, cardiovascular risks, and superior blood stress. NSAIDs can lessen blood waft to the kidneys, probably predominant to acute kidney damage, specially in sufferers with pre-present kidney contamination or those taking drug treatments that affect renal blood drift, which encompass angiotensin-changing enzyme (ACE) inhibitors or diuretics. The cardiovascular dangers associated with NSAIDs variety counting on the precise medicinal drug and affected person populace, however can include an accelerated risk of coronary heart assault, stroke, and coronary coronary heart failure. These dangers have to be cautiously weighed in the course of the capability advantages of NSAID use, particularly in sufferers with stated cardiovascular hazard elements.

To limit the dangers associated with NSAIDs, healthcare carriers need to conform with a affected character-targeted method that specializes inside the utilization of the bottom powerful dose for the shortest length viable. Additionally, patients should be carefully monitored for functionality side outcomes, and alternative ache control techniques ought to be taken into consideration in instances wherein the risks of NSAID use outweigh the benefits.

Opioid analgesics are a powerful elegance of medicinal drugs used to govern moderate to immoderate pain, collectively with neck pain. These medicinal drugs act on the mu, delta, and kappa opioid receptors within the primary involved gadget. By binding to those receptors, opioids lessen pain belief, offer remedy, and, in some instances, activate a experience of euphoria.

Some typically prescribed opioids for neck pain consist of hydrocodone (Vicodin, Lortab), oxycodone (OxyContin, Percocet), and tramadol (Ultram). These capsules are available in numerous formulations, such as immediate-launch, extended-release, and combination merchandise with different analgesics on the aspect of acetaminophen or NSAIDs. The preference of opioid and device is primarily based upon on elements which encompass the severity and period of ache, character affected person reaction, and the presence of any contraindications or functionality drug interactions.

While opioids may be effective for brief-time period alleviation of excessive neck pain, their use is related to enormous dangers. One of the number one worries with opioid use is the functionality for dependence, that could increase even though the medication is used as prescribed. Dependence takes region when the body turns into acquainted with the presence of the drug, critical to withdrawal signs and symptoms if the drug is discontinued.

In addition to dependence, opioids bring a hazard of dependancy. Addiction is a complex, continual mind illness characterised via manner of the usage of compulsive drug-trying to find conduct regardless of terrible effects. Factors which can make contributions to the development of opioid dependancy include genetics, environmental influences, and character mental elements along side a statistics of substance abuse or intellectual fitness issues.

The threat of overdose is a few unique enormous scenario with opioid use. Overdose can arise while a affected person takes an excessive amount of of the medication, both intentionally or by accident, ensuing in respiratory despair and, in excessive instances, dying. The threat of overdose is better in patients who combine opioids with one-of-a-kind foremost anxious device depressants, at the aspect of benzodiazepines or alcohol.

Due to those dangers, opioids need to be reserved for instances in which different ache management strategies have been vain or are contraindicated. When prescribing opioids for neck pain, healthcare carriers ought to carefully verify the affected person's chance elements for abuse, inclusive of private and circle of relatives statistics of substance abuse, highbrow health troubles, and previous records of opioid misuse. Providers must also take into account the use of risk mitigation strategies, collectively with prescription drug tracking applications and affected person-provider agreements, to restrict the ability for misuse and diversion.

When beginning opioid remedy for neck ache, the bottom effective dose ought to be used for the shortest period essential to attain pain relief and useful improvement. Healthcare agencies ought to cautiously display the affected man or woman's improvement and modify the dose as desired, considering factors which includes pain severity, realistic reputation, and the presence of any damaging outcomes. If a preference is made to stop opioid remedy, the dose should be tapered regularly to minimize withdrawal signs and symptoms and signs.

It is also vital for sufferers and healthcare carriers to be privy to the capability drug interactions amongst opioids and awesome medicinal drugs, further to any contraindications to opioid use. Some commonplace drug interactions encompass the mixture of opioids with benzodiazepines, that could growth the hazard of respiration melancholy, and the usage of opioids with positive antidepressants, that could result in a likely life-threatening circumstance known as serotonin syndrome.

Opioids may be an powerful choice for dealing with immoderate neck pain in pick out out out instances while used judiciously and with appropriate warning. Healthcare companies should carefully weigh the capability dangers and blessings of opioid treatment and rent strategies to restrict the hazard of dependence, dependancy, and overdose. Patients need to be educated about the proper use, storage, and disposal of opioids, further to the symptoms and signs and symptoms of overdose and the deliver of naloxone, an opioid antagonist that would contrary the results of an opioid overdose in emergency situations.

Chapter 7: Understanding Neck Pain

Any pain or pain felt inside the neck's vertebrae, discs amongst them, muscle companies, joints, or nerves is referred to as neck ache. For instance, stiffness or problems shifting your neck may additionally accompany ache. Neck ache introduced on thru nerve compression have to every so often be discovered thru numbness, tingling, or weak point in the hand or arm.

You need to first apprehend the essential structure of your spine and neck to understand your symptoms and signs and signs and symptoms and signs and symptoms and to be had remedy alternatives. This consists of being acquainted with the neck's many additives. You want to have preferred information of ways the ones components operate, that is, how they collaborate. The extra you recognize, the much less tough it is going to be an awesome way to provide an purpose of your unique condition for your clinical doctors and the relaxation of the clinical body of humans. It may even help you understand what they will be pronouncing approximately your precise problem.

The purpose of these records is that will help you recognize your neck ache trouble so that you can choose the exquisite path of movement to save you it.

Choose the remarkable path of motion to your harm, and hasten the healing machine.

Anatomy

Components of the Cervical Spine and Their Function

The cervical spine, this is the top a part of the spine, and the smooth tissues that surround it make up the bulk of the neck. Soft tissues consist of such things as blood arteries, nerves, muscular tissues, ligaments, and tendons. The Cervical backbone is made up of seven vertebrae. Your physician will often talk with those bones as C1 through C7. From certainly under the cranium to certainly above the thoracic spine is wherein the cervical spine starts offevolved offevolved. The spine serves two important functions:

to guard and preserve the spinal cord

to provide our our our bodies shape and stability simply so we are able to arise at once.

The 24 bones that unite to form the spinal column are referred to as vertebrae. Similar to how the bones of the skull shield the mind, the bones of the spine protect the spinal cord.

A community of nerves referred to as the spinal wire links the mind to the relaxation of the body.

Each vertebra has a big hole in its center. These holes line as a whole lot as create the spinal canal, a "bony tube" down which the spinal wire travels because of the truth the vertebrae are all fused. This bony tube shapes the spinal canal, which safeguards and helps the spinal twine.

After leaving the mind, the spinal twine passes through the spinal canal and ends on the tailbone. Along the way, it releases small nerves that pass through the foramen amongst every vertebra of the spine to go away. The cervical backbone's top component is wherein the nerves break out the backbone, and that they go to the arms and arms. The chest and belly are frequently wherein the thoracic spine's chest-place nerves go out the spine. The decrease spine, or lumbar spine, is in which the nerves that exit the spinal canal go together with the go together with the waft to the legs and feet.

To better apprehend how the numerous components of the spine work together, let's have a look at a spinal section. A spinal segment consists of vertebrae, an intervertebral disc, and nerve roots, one from every issue that "branch off."

in "the spine" The cervical vertebrae are the smallest vertebrae inside the backbone thinking about the reality that they do not assist as hundreds weight because the vertebrae inside the decrease again. One pair of spinal nerves emerges from every segment via the gap the numerous vertebrae. Pressure at the nerve roots is a not unusual purpose of pain that might reason numbness and ache inside the neck or decrease body.

A massive, round disc of connective tissue referred to as an intervertebral disc sits between vertebrae. From above, the intervertebral disc appears to have an annulus-normal outer ring and a nucleus pulposus-formed indoors. The disc's maximum effective place, the annulus, aids in retaining the spongy centre in the disc. By acting as a marvel absorber, the nucleus shields the bones from stress when twisting, leaping, or bearing weight.

A joint is created while or extra bones come together. Each vertebra's component joint is manufactured from overlapping bony protrusions referred to as side joints. The vertebrae are linked collectively like a sequence through issue joints, which give a cellular connection. Because they permit the neck to bend and flip, aspect joints are important. The spine is incredibly bendy irrespective of the restrained motion that each vertebra has on its very very personal.

Causes of Neck Pain

The disc is common of connective tissue, which in reality wears out as we age. Many of the issues that motive neck ache, but, are due to unusual placed on and pressure. This is known as intervertebral disc degeneration. Degeneration is regularly as a result of minor accidents that don't purpose pain on the time of the damage. These accidents gather over the years, and the bizarre placed on and tear can impair the connective tissue that makes up the disc. When the connective tissue is inclined, surprising strain, collectively with a whiplash movement, can with out issue injure the disc. Spondylolysis is a time period used to explain the complete gadget of disc degeneration. Your health practitioner might also additionally talk for your neck trouble as spondylolysis of the cervical backbone.

To sincerely realise neck pain, you want to first recognise the damage and tear and tear tool known as disc degeneration. This additionally will let you realize what can appear to the neck even as there may be a unexpected damage that motives ache and dysfunction.

DDD stands for Degenerative Disc Disease.

Compare a spinal phase to 2 vanilla wafers (the "vertebrae") and a marshmallow (the "disc") to higher understand disc degeneration. Imagine a sparkling marshmallow sandwiched amongst wafers. The marshmallow yields or "squishes out" while the wafers are pressed together tightly. Assume you depart the marshmallow out for every week and it starts offevolved to dry. It's now not pretty as spongy whilst pressed a number of the wafers. If you press difficult sufficient, the marshmallow's exterior can also rip or split. Assume you had the marshmallow out for a month.

It might most probably be so dried out that it is probably inflexible and simply skinny, with little "surprise soaking up" homes.

The disc loses a number of its water content cloth cloth and, as a forestall stop result, a number of its surprise-soaking up abilties as we age. The earliest changes in the disc, much like the marshmallow, are tears in the outer ring of the disc, called the annulus. Tears in the annulus can arise with out inflicting any signs and signs. As a stop end result, you could now not observe when they show up or what brought on them. These tears are healed thru the formation of scar tissue. Scar tissue is more fragile than ordinary tissue. Repeated injuries and tears cause the disc to wear down faster. The water content material fabric of the disc decreases because it wears. It grows a bargain much less "spongy" through the years, subsequently dropping its capacity to act as a surprise absorber.

As the disc deteriorates, it starts offevolved to crumble. The hollow between each vertebra narrows. The disintegrate additionally has an effect on how the factor joints inside the rear of the spine "line up." The shift inside the manner the bones wholesome together, like each different joint inside the frame,

generates irrelevant stress on the articular cartilage. The easy, colorful material that covers the ends of the bones in any joint is referred to as articular cartilage. This aberrant pressure produces placed on and tear arthritis (osteoarthritis) of the aspect joints over the years.

Around the disc and element joints, bone spurs can broaden. It is idea that immoderate mobility in a spinal segment motives bone spurs to amplify. Spinal stenosis is because of the formation of bone spurs around the nerves of the spine.

Stenosis of the backbone

Spinal stenosis is a narrowing of the spinal canal that reasons nerve roots to be compressed. This constriction is maximum not unusual inside the neck or decrease returned.

Pain inside the neck, lower once more, or legs is not unusual in human beings with spinal stenosis. The ache is regularly exacerbated thru movement, but, posing the neck in a particular manner can from time to time alleviate the discomfort.

Spinal stenosis is typically because of osteoarthritis. Spinal tumours, begin abnormalities, and Paget's disease are some of the possibility reasons of this illness.

Types of Neck pain

Muscle tenseness

When a patient complains of a stiff neck, a "muscle stress" of the neck is a common analysis. In some instances, this may be a "muscle strain" or "pulled muscle" affecting the muscle companies surrounding the spinal column within the neck. Muscle spasm, alternatively, is a not unusual signal that could get up on the same time as exclusive components of the neck are injured. In muscular strain issues, super smooth tissues of the neck, which includes the disc, ligaments across the spinal segment, and muscle corporations, may be affected. If any of those systems is harmed, similar signs and symptoms and signs can also emerge.

Mechanical Causes of Neck Pain

A continual neck pain this is felt regularly in the neck may be due to arthritis inside the cervical backbone's facet joints and degenerative disc degeneration. Mechanical pain is a term used by clinical doctors to provide an cause of this shape of suffering. This time period is used as it worsens with improved neck use and looks to be due to mechanical additives of the cervical backbone that permit us to transport our heads up and down and round.

The nerves producing this ache are neither pinched or infected. Inflamed thing joints and a degenerating disc appear like the property of the ache. When we circulate our heads with our necks, the disc and element joints turn out to be extra infected, causing the muscular tissues surrounding the cervical spine to spasm. A spasm influences the muscular tissues within the same manner that a cramp does. Muscle cramping subsequently creates pain. The spasm is due to the body's try to prevent the cervical backbone from transferring.

Compression of the Nerves Radiculopathy of the Cervical Spine

A nerve root descends into the arm after leaving the cervical spine and spinal cord. Each neuron alongside the pathway gives electric powered impulses to particular muscle companies, permitting movement of a phase of the arm or hand further to sensation (feeling) to a patch of pores and skin at the shoulder and arm. When a nerve is infected or compressed, whether or not via a bone spur or a portion of the intervertebral disc, it can not function well. This manifests as muscle weak spot, numbness inside the pores and pores and skin wherein the nerve passes, or pain in that place. Cervical radiculopathy is the scientific term for this disorder.

Discomfort in the nerves

It is pretty difficult to outline neck nerve pain. Each vertebra has one or more spinal twine-derived nerves that exit the body. Inflammation or anatomical damage at these go out net websites can squeeze, impinge, or aggravate the nerve roots, resulting in ache that may be mild or excessive, transitory or chronic, and located through burning or a pins-and-needles sensation. Depending on the nerve implicated, pain might probable go down the arm or maybe into the hand, and it may be exacerbated through each preferred or specialized motion.

How to Avoid Neck Pain

Change the pillow.

There are numerous approaches to help and simplicity your neck while you sleep, so selecting the most effective that works satisfactory for you may take a few trial and errors. In cutting-edge, it is most widely recognized to apply a pillow that maintains unbiased spinal alignment at the same time as helping and keeping your neck's natural curve.

As frequently as you could, try and sleep in your decrease returned.

Generally speaking, dozing in your once more is the amazing characteristic to provide your whole backbone a proper relaxation. Some neck pain sufferers discover it beneficial to sleep on their backs with a pillow beneath every arm inside the wish that retaining up each arm can also relieve neck pain.

Some human beings with spinal stenosis or arthritis may moreover discover that it's miles greater snug to sleep barely stepped forward, in order that they purchase an adjustable mattress or regulate their bed with a foam wedge cushion.

Make superb the show display in your pc is at eye stage.

Sit down in the the front of the pc effects as you shut up your eyes. Your eyes should be at the pinnacle zero.33 of your pc show at the same time as you first open them. If You become conscious that you ought to raise your show and appearance down.

It is usually pretty useful to attach your pc to an outside reveal or show because of the reality laptops require you to hunch to appearance the display display display screen.

When texting, try to keep away from using your neck.

Your neck will enjoy brilliant pressure if you text or spend some of time searching down at a cellular cellular phone or other cellular device.

The introduced pressure in your neck's joints, ligaments, and discs over time may also additionally hasten the onset of degenerative adjustments. By lifting the cellular telephone or mobile tool to eye degree, restricting the length of time spent texting, resting your hands and tool on a pillow, and pausing regularly, texting neck pressure may be avoided.

Employ a headset.

Avoid leaning to at least one problem or resting your telephone in the crook of your neck in case you often talk at the cellular telephone.

An earpiece, headset, or extraordinary arms-unfastened device is a first rate manner to talk at the cellphone while not having to keep it uncomfortably. A greater current-day system is likewise available that you may placed on round your neck all day.

Simplest bodily activities for Neck Pain

superior neck warm temperature

Start via retaining your neck right away. Bring your chin slightly in advance. Take a step once more to in which you have been after protective for 5 seconds. Please say that ten extra times.

neck elongation

Slowly flip your head lower returned, dealing with up, without arching your lower again. Hold for a whole of 5 seconds. Return to the beginning. Try this exercise to help your neck experience lots much less tight at the same time as running.

turning your neck

Start via using searching at straight away earlier. Turn your head slowly to the left. Once you have held for ten seconds, keep on from in that you left off. Then slowly turn your head to the alternative facet. The function must be held for ten seconds. Return to the start. Repeat ten instances. This is a top notch place of work exercising when you have to keep your head immobile for a long term, like at the same time as the use of a computer. To save you neck pain, repeat this exercise each half-hour.

On the extender's component

Start by way of the use of way of observing right away in advance. Turn your head slowly to the left. Strenuously squeeze your neck muscle groups at the identical time as the usage of your left hand as resistance. Take a step lower returned to in which you had been after keeping for 5 seconds. Next, softly incline the opportunity aspect in conjunction with your head. Hold for an entire of five seconds. Return to the begin. Repeat ten times. This is a amazing place of work exercising when you have to hold your head immobile for a long time, like even as the use of a pc. To prevent neck ache, repeat this workout each half of-hour.

shoulders slumping

Start by means of the use of gazing proper away in advance. Raise every shoulders step by step. Take a step decrease returned to in which you were after holding for 5 seconds. Repeat ten times. This is a tremendous place of work exercise if you have to maintain your head immobile for a long term, like while using a pc. To save you neck ache, repeat this workout each half of-hour.

willing to the front

Start by using the use of using looking immediately in advance. Put your chin slowly in your chest. Take a step decrease again to wherein you've got been after defensive for five seconds. Repeat ten times. This serves for instance of

This is a terrific exercising to do on the identical time as running, particularly when you have to keep your head regular loads, along with at the same time as using a pc. To prevent neck pain, repeat this exercising every half-hour.

Continuous Stretching

Allow your head to sag in the direction of your shoulder even as sitting up right away. As confirmed, you may follow pressure collectively with your hand. Alternatively, you can use the opportunity hand to grip your chair. After keeping for 30 seconds, carry out 3 repetitions.

Presses of Resistance

Maintain a independent head function constantly. Squeeze your head for five seconds in each of the ensuing positions in advance than letting skip. A hand on the brow will display flexion. Extend your hand in the decrease lower back of your head in the the front of you.

Chapter 8: Headache Explain

A headache is characterized thru way of ache or ache within the head or face. The type of headache, its region, intensity, and frequency all range. The thoughts tissue can not enjoy ache as it lacks ache-touchy nerve fibres. A headache, but, may also originate everywhere inside the head, in conjunction with the subsequent:

a community of nerves that runs for the duration of the scalp

mouth, throat, and facial nerves

muscle companies inside the shoulders, neck, and head

Blood vessels cowl the thoughts's ground and base.

Types Of Headache

Migraine

This shape of headache consists of extra signs and symptoms and symptoms and signs and symptoms similarly to ache. Photophobia, disorientation, and specific visible issues are talents of migraines in addition to nausea and vomiting. Even migraines extend over time. However, now not all and sundry moves on to the subsequent level. The stages of a migraine headache are as follows:

a traumatic or early period.

Before the headache, it can take hours or days for a intellectual or behavioural change to take location.

The air of mystery's section has commenced.

Before the headache, there might have been a string of visible, sensory, or motor troubles. Those who're affected may also have eye distortion, hallucinations, numbness, trouble speakme, and muscle weak point.

The headache's stage.

There also can be throbbing pain on one or every elements of the pinnacle in addition to the headache. Typical signs and symptoms embody fatigue, anxiety, sensitivity to light, and melancholy.

the spot in which a choice is probably.

The ache disappears proper now, but it may get replaced with exhaustion, impatience, or despair.

It's tough for me to pay interest proper now.

Some people regain their power after an attack, whilst others do not.

complications resulting with the aid of tension

The most everyday type of headache is the Tension headache Tension headaches are often delivered on via stress and sore muscle companies. The following list includes some of the most time-commemorated warning symptoms of hysteria complications:

A moderate headache first takes region.

Both aspects of the top usually harm.

The stupid ache is sort of a vice or ring across the cranium. Additionally, the lower back of the neck or the cranium may be affected.

The ache is tolerable, regardless of how mild or severe it's miles. Rarely do tension headaches result in nausea, dizziness, or a worry of mild called photophobia.

occasional complications

Cluster headache symptoms and symptoms and signs and signs and symptoms and signs and symptoms embody those indexed beneath:

Cluster complications commonly appear in waves over the course of several weeks or months.

Cluster headache signs and symptoms and signs and symptoms and signs and signs and symptoms encompass the ones indexed beneath:

a headache that looks on one element of the pinnacle and inside the back of 1 eye.

A watery, red, and painful eye condition can be located via a constricted pupil and drooping lids.

coughing or congestion, puffy eyes

Straight brows are present.

Causes of Headache

People often lay their palms on both component in their heads even as affected by a great, agonising headache and exclaim, "I sense like my mind is pushing to get out, so it feels higher to keep it in." This sensation effects in the incorrect impact that the thoughts's increase is generating pain. Contrary to well-known perception, mind tissue does not revel in pain within the identical way that pores and skin or exceptional organs do. Because the brain is enclosed in a hard, shielding shell, it has now not advanced to reply to touch or stress sensations within the equal manner that exclusive, more uncovered components of our our bodies have. A mind health care provider may also additionally do surgical procedure on a aware affected individual whilst reducing thoughts tissue without the affected individual feeling the knife.

The activation or stimulation of natural tissues which includes the pores and pores and skin, neck or bone joints, sinuses, blood vessels, or muscle organizations causes headaches. When a mind tumour has advanced to the point wherein it's far inflicting bone damage, blockading blood vessels, or urgent on nerves, ache regularly seems an entire lot later. Neck issues, similarly to complications, can reason complications, and ache within the neck and all over again of the pinnacle often extending to the attention. Sinus

Recurrent complications are not often due to contamination or infection (which frequently takes location at the side of an hypersensitivity). According to Roger Cady and Curtis Schneider of the Headache Care Center in Springfield, Missouri, 25 to 30% of migraineurs enjoy nasal signs and signs inside the path in their common migraine attacks, and almost ninety eight percent of folks who concept that they'd sinus complications had migraines.

Migraine and tension-kind headaches are the most traditional forms of persistent headaches. A migraine is an intermittent headache that happens as soon as a month or times every week and lasts 8 to 12 hours on every occasion. Migraine is normally described as a severe, one-sided headache that interferes with every day sports activities. Nausea and sensitivity to fragrance, moderate, and sound are amongst viable thing consequences. Tension headaches can maintain for severa days and come to be greater frequent as time passes. The soreness is commonly defined as a moderate pressure ache that does not save you day by day sports on each aspects of the pinnacle. These types of complications are resulting from internal or outside factors which incorporates pressure, loss of sleep, fasting, or hormonal adjustments. When high best cues are supplied to the mind, it prompts.

to deliver pain indicators to the thoughts's ache centres, which reasons the meningeal blood vessels surrounding the thoughts to swell and release numerous chemical messengers along with serotonin and norepinephrine. This boom motives an boom in blood go with the flow, that may make blood vessels at the aspect of the top greater visible and painful. When the encircling nerves come to be stretched out due to blood vessel increase, they send signs to the trigeminal device, a area of the mind that relays ache indicators to the pinnacle and face. Pain that appears to be "sinus"-like is most usually due to trigeminal tool activation and is felt all through the face and eyes. The trigeminal system moreover communicates with the top phase of the cervical spinal cord, that might reason neck muscle spasms, and the hypothalamus, part of the thoughts related to meals desires.

Headache drug treatments have a difficult time operating as speedy because the complete headache pathway is lively. Rami Burstein's ultra-modern Harvard University research has time and again showed that taking painkillers early in a headache episode is essential for his or her effectiveness in mice and people. Migraine sufferers often describe that their headaches start as a throbbing sensation in advance than escalating to greater sensitive pores and pores and skin. Pain may be due to allodynia, or heightened pores and skin sensitivity, even as combing one's hair, placing on jewelry, or wearing eyeglasses. It may additionally purpose scalp inflammation and "painful" hair. Headache treatments come to be drastically much less effective after allodynia happens. By meticulously documenting headache symptoms and signs and symptoms and symptoms and symptoms in a diary, it's far viable to understand whilst allodynia occurs and while to take drugs that provide the most comfort.

Even although maximum chronic headaches are not because of essential illnesses, a massive alternate in headache pattern, the discontinuation of a formerly effective remedy, or the emergence of latest health troubles further to the headache have to purpose a go to to the medical physician for an assessment.

How to Avoid Headache

Headaches are a common disorder that influences nearly truly every body in a few unspecified time within the destiny of their lives. While a few complications are best mildly bothersome, others may be in reality incapacitating.

Many over-the-counter and prescription treatments are available to treat headache signs and symptoms, however, fine drug treatments might also have unfavourable component consequences if used excessively. Taking ache relievers greater than 3 times in step with week can result in rebound headaches. Acetaminophen overuse has been related to liver harm, whilst ibuprofen and aspirin overuse can damage the kidneys and worsen the stomach.

Take the subsequent movements to decrease the risk of complications truly if you be stricken by way of common complications.

1. Drink a whole lot of water

According to investigate, dehydration can purpose each migraines and anxiety complications. Dehydration can also produce symptoms along with fear and exhaustion, that can irritate headaches.

It is easy to become dehydrated with out even recognizing it. Attempt to eat seventy eight-a hundred oz.. Of water each day. Check out those water-consumption-boosting pointers if you're having trouble staying hydrated.

2. Consume Magnesium Supplements

Magnesium is a mineral that aids in muscle and nerve characteristic. Magnesium deficiency has been related to muscle spasms, cramping, and migraines. Consume food immoderate in magnesium, together with leafy greens, legumes, nuts, and seeds. Consider taking a magnesium supplement to beautify your food plan. Remember that magnesium dietary dietary supplements can motive digestive troubles (which include diarrhoea) in some humans, so begin with a low dose.

three. Get Enough Rest

The exquisite of your sleep could have pretty some consequences on your fitness. Sleep deprivation has been related to immune tool disorder, melancholy, weight benefit, horrible mind feature, or maybe coronary coronary coronary heart illness. Lack of sleep is regularly the purpose of Headaches. According to 1 have a study, those who received much less than six hours of sleep steady with night time had higher headaches.

If you've got problem snoozing, start working on enhancing your sleep hygiene right away.

If critical, see a clinical health practitioner approximately capsules that might aid inside the treatment of insomnia.

four. Avoid Certain Food Ingredients

Certain meals components were associated with complications in sure men and women. Among those are nitrates and nitrites, which is probably preservatives regularly discovered in processed meats like warm puppies, bloodless cuts, and bacon. When purchasing for processed meat, look for chemical substances like sodium nitrate, sodium nitrite, potassium nitrate, or potassium nitrite.

MSG and aspartame are more meals chemical substances which have been related to migraines. Make it a addiction to have a observe component labels so you can keep away from devices that can cause complications.

5. Limit Alcohol Consumption

Alcohol has been diagnosed as a migraine cause in a single-1/three of migraine sufferers. Tension complications and cluster headaches have moreover been related to it.

The form of alcohol you drink also can boom your chances of having a headache. Red wine, as an instance, is the

The most not unusual alcoholic beverage is hooked up with anxiety and cluster headaches. If you get complications after ingesting pink wine, try switching to white wine or a few other drink.

Home Remedies for Headache

To cope with or save you migraine attacks, more than a few medicinal drugs are available. Additional symptom treatment may be provided with the useful resource of natural remedies.

Ten all-herbal migraine remedy and prevention strategies are indexed underneath.

Acupuncture

Thomas Barwick/Getty Images is the photographer.

Applying stress on specific frame additives is referred to as acupressure. Pain relief is the purpose of activating these regions.

Both specialists and amateurs can examine acupressure at home. However, it's far tremendous to speak with an expert earlier than you start.

Headaches can be efficiently treated the use of acupressure on the LI-4 aspect, that is situated maximum of the bottom of the left thumb and the index finger. Apply company round pressure with the opposing hand for 5 mins at the LI-4 element to relieve headache signs and symptoms.

Diet

It's viable that converting one's weight loss plan will help someone avoid migraine assaults. This is because of the fact, for some people, superb meals ought to probably initiate migraines.

Some normal food that reason migraines embody the subsequent:

cooked meats

alcohol

caffeinated chocolate

Oils for aromatherapy

The lavender crucial oil has the functionality to address headaches, strain, and anxiety. A 2021 literature compare determined that eleven extremely good styles of vital oils incorporate substances that could reduce the symptoms and symptoms of migraines. Among them are basil, chamomile, lavender, and peppermint.

These effects appear to be supported through advantageous clinical investigations. One hundred forty four members in a 2020 triple-blind examine that used basil oil as a topical treatment observed a discount in migraine symptom severity and frequency.

To research which important oils work first-rate and the way to apply them, more scientific studies are essential.

It is essential to be conscious that a few critical oils might also moreover pose a chance to youngsters, humans who have allergies, and ladies who're pregnant or breastfeeding. Do now not use them without first speaking in your physician.

Only a diffuser want to be used to inhale essential oils. Before utilizing topically, continuously dilute with corporation oil at a safe awareness.

Ginger A 2021 evaluation Three instructional studies determined that ginger powder emerge as every steady and effective for alleviating migraines. When in comparison to control groups, it considerably lessened ache after hours. Ginger can assist with nausea and vomiting as well.

While ginger can also have advantages, there may be moreover a risk that it may intervene with or have negative outcomes. For example, warfarin customers may be extra inclined. A reliable bleeding supply. Make an appointment with a physician earlier than attempting it.

Stress control

Stress is a regarded migraine purpose for 7 out of 10 sufferers. It could probably even start a vicious cycle in which stress will growth migraine pain, which then reasons each other migraine.

When viable, it is in truth useful to stay a long way from situations that might be annoying. It is probably beneficial to find retailers at the facet of journaling, exercising, and meditation. Additional techniques for reducing stress embody taking a warm temperature bath, taking note of tune, or schooling breathing physical sports. Stress manipulate training are first rate to certain human beings.

6 Yoga

A previous take a look at from 2014 Trusted Source as compared everyday yoga workout to the equal vintage migraine treatment. The have a examine's findings showed that the yoga agency felt greater consolation than the business enterprise receiving cutting-edge hospital therapy. For six weeks, contributors did yoga 5 days every week.

7. Biofeedback remedy.

A shape of treatment known as biofeedback teaches sufferers a way to deliberately manage bodily processes.

Most of the time, human beings are asleep. For example, a person should likely learn how to unwind their muscle tissue.

Users can recognize tight muscle mass with the use of a small device that receives statistics from sensors on the targeted muscles and materials real-time comments on muscle anxiety.

Sensors located alongside the jawline, shoulders, or trapezius muscle businesses also can assist humans purpose the muscle organizations which may be responsible for migraine signs and symptoms.

8. Acupuncture.

To achieve particular effects, a practitioner puts needles into positive frame regions within the route of acupuncture remedy. Similar to acupressure, it.

A targeted systematic assessment of the literature that evaluated the efficacy of acupuncture for the remedy of migraines have turn out to be done in 2020. The scientists determined that acupuncture have become a constant and green remedy choice for human beings with migraine complications.

They did, but, point out that severa studies had been of low extremely good and that extra credible research modified into needed. Anyone who desires to attempt it want to

A official and certified expert need to administer acupuncture.

9. Rubdown treatment

Stress and migraine symptoms and signs and symptoms and symptoms may be decreased with the aid of massaging the neck and shoulder muscle groups. Stress comfort from massage also can be feasible.

A character would possibly possibly advantage from getting a rub down from a expert. Anyone interested by self-massaging their manner out of a migraine can roll a clean tennis ball round their shoulders and again on the same time as leaning up in opposition to a wall.

10. Minerals encompass magnesium.

Menstrual migraine headaches or migraine aura can be added on with the aid of manner of a deficiency within the crucial mineral magnesium.

According to a look at, supplementing with magnesium may also moreover help a few human beings lessen the frequency of seizures.

Consult your scientific medical doctor in advance than taking this complement, specifically when you have any other health troubles.

Exercises for Headache Relief

Chin Tucks

This exercise is one in every of my favourites to provide to my sufferers. The majority of those who sit down at desks in workplaces are guilty of slouching over and rounding their shoulders. A awesome way to align your head, neck, and shoulders is to tuck your chin.

Sit up right away, buttocks in opposition to the seat decrease returned, and lower again flat against the chair another time. Without cocking your head, decorate your chin in your throat. To provide a evaluation, I like to say, "Give your self a double chin without tilting the cranium down." For five seconds, hold this posture earlier than letting flow into. 10 instances every hour, repeat.

The Upper Trapezius Stretch

When we are sitting, our shoulders have a propensity to hike up, which reasons our top trapezius muscles to become hectic and rigid. You can stretch your shoulders to assist them end up extra bendy.

Sit or stand without delay to begin. Your proper ear have to be close to your right shoulder. Make fine your left shoulder does now not hike up in the path of your ear, nor does your proper shoulder climb up within the route of your ear. Holding this role, enhance your proper hand and

above the skull's left aspect. Once you feel a slight tug along the left shoulder and neck, slowly tilt the top to the proper. After 30 seconds, keep this posture earlier than moving lower once more to the midline. Repetition of this exercise at the possibility element. Repeat 2-three times on each difficulty.

Cat-Cow Stretch

This is a tremendous way to growth decrease again and neck mobility for those who spend loads of time sitting at art work.

On the floor, get down on your arms and knees alongside aspect your wrists below your shoulders. Starting with the backbone neutral, the returned flat, and the stomach muscle groups shriveled. Take a massive breath in and lift your head and tailbone on the same time as arching your decrease back. Then, exhale at the identical time as bringing your chin for your chest, pulling your tailbone in, pressing your abdominals into your backbone, and doing the identical to your tailbone. Change amongst those two positions numerous instances at the same time as inhaling and exhaling. Keep going for a minute.

Move your head backward and forward in motion.

This is particularly beneficial if you revel in stiffness on your neck at the same time as tilting your head from left to proper.

Start by manner of way of assuming a right away posture. Look over your right shoulder at the side of your head have come to be to the proper for ten seconds, or till you can not hold this posture. Repeat on the alternative aspect, then get once more to your beginning role. Repeat three times.

Scalp Retraction

At work, do you become bored? The best workout to carry out whilst seated at paintings is this. It lets in prevent the in advance head and rounded shoulders posture that is everyday inside the administrative center.

First, permit the tops of your shoulders lighten up. Next, picture a tennis ball amongst your shoulder blades and pinch them collectively to overwhelm the "ball." Repeat 10 instances an hour.

Chapter 9: Arm Ache Defined

There are severa causes of arm pain. Wear and tear, overuse, injury, a pinched nerve, and certain health problems collectively with rheumatoid arthritis or fibromyalgia are examples of these. Arm pain can arise quick or frequently, relying on the purpose.

Arm ache can be because of issues with the muscle agencies, bones, tendons, ligaments, or nerves. It may also be related to problems with the shoulders, elbows, and wrists. Arm pain is often due to a hassle in your neck or top spine. Arm ache, especially pain radiating into your left arm, can be a sign of a coronary coronary heart attack.

Causes of Arm pain

Any a part of your body can also need to turn out to be uncomfortable. Pain might also follow an damage, it truly is to be predicted, but it is able to additionally originate from another area. For example, ache in the fingers and hands would probable broaden without an damage for a few reasons. Because you operate your palms and fingers for such numerous activities, alongside aspect writing, typing, and carrying items inner your home, pain may be frightening and keep you from getting the assignment achieved.

The most standard reasons for arm pain are listed beneath.

ordinary motion

The muscular tissues, ligaments, and tendons to your arm or hand can also get strained if the identical motion is over and over finished with quick interruptions. As a forestall cease end result of repetitive movement in the arm or hand, not unusual issues that increase encompass:

Tendonitis

Inflammation of the tendons, the fibrous fibres that join your muscle agencies in your bones, is referred to as tendonitis. Any tendon for your arm or hands also can become infected in case you carry out the same pass time and again.

Tennis elbow, for example, is added on with the resource of the usage of the ordinary again-and-forth motion of your forearm in some unspecified time in the future of play. But no longer pleasant tennis gamers can growth tennis elbow; painters, butchers, and plumbers can as nicely. You may be at risk of irritation in case you glide your computer mouse constantly for the duration of the day.

CTS, or carpal tunnel syndrome

The median nerve, which could offer feeling to the thumb, index, center, and ring hands, becomes compressed because it travels through the carpal tunnel to your wrist, foremost to carpal tunnel syndrome, a not unusual purpose of hand and arm ache. The tendons to your wrist might also swell due to repetitive interest, inclusive of that determined on an meeting line, that could motive pain and nerve compression.

By changing your recurring, you might be capable of save you the pain that repetitive movement reasons on your fingers and hands. At CHOICE Discomfort & Rehabilitation Center, our experts will let you in figuring out the manner to alter your motions to lessen soreness.

Age-associated natural wear and tear

Wisdom might also moreover come with age, but joint health is likewise affected. As the cartilage between your joints deteriorates through the years, allowing the bones to rub in opposition to each different, you could have pain for your palms or fingers. Osteoarthritis is some different call for this circumstance.

However, it goes beyond your joints and cartilage. The rotator cuff, a fixed of tendons that keep your arm and shoulder in place, can also get torn because of tissue degeneration. Your capability to use your arm may be hampered via shoulder ache from a rotator cuff tear that radiates down your arm. Degeneration usually moreover affects your dominant hand.

It might be your neck.

Something other than your extremities may be the supply of your arm or hand pain. Your neck conditions like a herniated disc or spinal stenosis may be accountable for the sensations jogging down your arm and into your fingers. The nerves that transmit signs and symptoms down your arm and into your arms have to get angry thru those situations. You want to have your neck tested when you have tingling or numbness for your arms or hands.

That weird boom on your wrist

A ganglion cyst, a noncancerous development filled with the lubricating fluid for your joint, can be the deliver of that bizarre lump. Although commonly no longer bothersome, those little lumps have the capability to be painful in the occasion that they push within the route of a nerve. The cyst can be treated with immobilisation, fluid drainage, or an entire cystectomy.

terrible fall

Even in case you did no longer smash any bones, a awful fall can injure your arm or hand's tendons, ligaments, or muscle tissue, which can be painful. You have a tendency to rest, use over the counter pain relievers, and practice an ice percentage to your self at the same time as staying in. Understanding the underlying cause of your ache, however, will let you get the exquisite care for a fast restoration. For example, in case you ruptured your rotator cuff after a difficult cope with in football exercise, not receiving the ideal care should make the damage worse.

Arm and hand soreness can rise up for hundreds one-of-a-type reasons. Finding the reason of your ache can be helpful.

The first-rate possible care is probably given to you. To discover what is inflicting your pain, supply CHOICE Pain & Rehabilitation Center a call right away or time table an appointment on line.

How to Avoid Arm pain

1. Warming up in advance than workout or acting repetitive tasks to save you anxiety at the muscle mass and tendons inside the fingers is one technique to keep away from arm pain.

2. Take commonplace breaks from repetitious jobs to permit your fingers to rest.

3. Maintain right posture even as sitting or standing to keep away from tension at the neck and shoulders, that could result in arm ache.

4. Lift heavy objects with unique shape to avoid arm and shoulder harm.

5. Stretch on a each day basis to preserve your arm muscle groups and tendons flexible and reduce your chance of damage.

6. To avoid damage, use supportive shoes and use suitable device whilst participating in sports activities sports.

7. Maintain a healthy weight to prevent stress at the arm and shoulder joints.

eight. Avoid smoking as it reduces blood go along with the flow to the arms and will increase the hazard of infection and damage.

nine. If your career goals repetitive arm motions, speak ergonomic alternatives alongside facet your company, in conjunction with adjustable workstations or gadgets designed to alleviate pressure at the palms and shoulders.

Natural Remedy for Arm Pain

You can try these clean, natural domestic remedies for arm pain to eliminate arm ache fast.

1. Cold Massage

One of the best treatments for arm pain is a cold compress. The cool temperature will numb the tissue within the affected place, relieving ache. This furthermore allows to minimise infection.

Wrap an ice dice in a towel and wrap it over your arm.

Keep the towel in area for 15 minutes.

For a few days, repeat this technique each day.

2. Ascension

You can lessen arm pain via raising the troubled arm. Elevation promotes adequate blood flow into within the arm region and speeds up the recovery method.

When you're resting or slumbering, location one or two pillows under your arm.

This technique will enhance blood go with the flow.

three. The Hot Compress

A heat compress allows alleviate arm aches. This treatment is exceptional effective after forty eight hours from the time the harm or pain began out.

Fill a bath with heat water and immerse your arm for 10-15 mins.

Use this method at least instances a day.

four. Rest

Resting your hand correctly will assist to restore soft tissue damage due to minor ache. To alleviate soreness and infection, region your fingers on a clean pillow. Allow the arm to rest for seventy hours without wearing out any intense activities.

5. Therapeutic massage

Massage is any other powerful home cure for arm ache. It will aid inside the remedy of pressure within the hurting area.

A tablespoon of mustard oil or coconut oil is warmed.

Apply the heated oil to the sore spot.

Gently rubdown the arm to increase blood glide.

Repeat this a couple of times in the course of the day.

6. Turmeric is a spice.

Turmeric additionally may be used to address arm pain. Curcumin, a chemical positioned in turmeric, has anti inflammatory and antioxidant traits that assist to lessen swelling and ache.

Make a paste with 2 teaspoons of turmeric powder and 1 teaspoon of coconut oil.

Apply this paste to the aching arm.

Use this technique at the least instances a day.

7. Ginger

Ginger is some different beneficial remedy for arm ache. It includes antioxidants and anti inflammatory trends that could help to lessen any shape of contamination. Ginger promotes blood motion and hurries up the healing system.

You can eat 3 glasses of ginger tea constant with day.

8. Cayenne Pepper consists of a chemical known as capsaicin, which has analgesic and anti-inflammatory capabilities that useful aid within the comfort of arm ache.

Combine 12 teaspoons of cayenne pepper and 1 tablespoon lukewarm olive oil.

Apply it to the affected area and gently massage it for 30 seconds.

9. Apple Cider Vinegar

Another first rate remedy for arm pain is apple cider vinegar. It possesses alkalizing and anti-inflammatory tendencies, which beneficial aid in the cut price of swelling and ache.

To your bathtub water, upload 2 cups of uncooked, unfiltered apple cider vinegar.

Spend 1/2 of-hour soaking in it.

Use this technique every day.

10. Lavender vital oil

Lavender oil is an vital oil used to calm tired muscular tissues. It will relieve arm pain and contamination.

In your tub water, add 5 drops of lavender oil.

Soak your arm for 1/2-hour in it.

11. Magnesium Foods

Magnesium aids in muscular contraction and nerve interest, consequently it is able to help relieve arm pain.

Consume magnesium-rich meals which encompass beans, nuts, green leafy vegetables, entire grains, and so on.

Chapter 10: Pain Control

The clinical place of knowledge that specializes in minimising and controlling pain, especially chronic pain, is referred to as ache control. It includes pretty some treatments and techniques aimed at lowering pain, improving characteristic and splendid of lifestyles, and addressing the foundation causes of ache. A type of ailments, collectively with arthritis, most cancers, fibromyalgia, migraines, and again pain, can be dealt with with ache control. Medication, physical therapy, acupuncture, nerve blocks, and one in every of a kind techniques may be used as treatment. The purpose of pain manipulate is to help patients live more with out problems and have a better notable of life on the identical time as lowering the dangers associated with prolonged-time period ache drug utilization.

Pain management is an interdisciplinary technique that consists of a multidisciplinary organisation of healthcare experts which encompass physicians, nurses, physical therapists, occupational therapists, psychologists, and distinctive experts. The enterprise collaborates to create a completely unique remedy plan for each affected individual based totally totally on their precise goals and dreams.

Pain treatment strategies are categorized into types: pharmacological and non-pharmacological. Medications which encompass opioids, nonsteroidal anti inflammatory tablets (NSAIDs), and antidepressants are utilized in pharmacological remedy. Physical treatment, acupuncture, massage remedy, cognitive-behavioural remedy, and exclusive interventions are examples of non-pharmacological treatments.

Pain control is specially critical for those who be bothered via continual pain, that is described as ache that lasts more than 3 months. Chronic pain can harm a person's splendid of lifestyles and might bring about depression, tension, and exceptional intellectual troubles. Pain manipulate can help to alleviate continual pain, boom characteristic, and beautify regular properly-being.

Overall, ache control is an important thing of healthcare which can help people live extra successfully and revel in a better incredible of life. If you're in pain, you have to talk over together together with your healthcare professional to become aware about the excellent course of treatment in your precise necessities.

Importance of pain manipulate

Pain manipulate is critical as it allows human beings to control their ache and live a higher lifestyles. Pain can be incapacitating, interfering with each day sports activities sports, jobs, and relationships. Effective ache control can help to relieve pain, increase function, and enhance popular well-being.

Chronic ache, especially, has been verified to harm a person's highbrow fitness, principal to disappointment, anxiety, and one in every of a type highbrow troubles. Pain manage can help to relieve those signs at the equal time as furthermore enhancing elegant highbrow health.

Furthermore, pain manage is crucial due to the fact it may lessen the need for delivered intrusive treatments like surgical procedure. Individuals who nicely manage their pain can be able to avoid surgical procedure or unique greater invasive measures.

Overall, ache management is an critical element of healthcare. It consists of an interdisciplinary technique wherein a group of healthcare specialists collaborates to layout a remedy plan.

Each affected man or woman gets a very particular remedy plan. If you're in ache, you need to speak over along with your healthcare professional to pick out the pleasant path of remedy in your unique requirements.

Dietary answer for Arm ache

There are nutritional alternatives that might help control pain in addition to medicinal remedy. Here are a few illustrations:

1. Anti-inflammatory weight loss program: An anti-inflammatory diet plan consists of food that assist the body's efforts to minimise contamination, that could aggravate ache. Leafy vegetables, berries, fatty fish, almonds, and olive oil are a few anti-inflammatory meals examples.

2. Omega-three fatty acids: Omega-three fatty acids are widely recognized for his or her capacity to fight contamination and decrease ache. Walnuts, flaxseeds, chia seeds, and fatty fish are examples of food excessive in omega-3s.

three. Turmeric: A spice having anti-inflammatory traits, curcumin is decided in turmeric. Including turmeric in meals or taking a complement containing curcumin can also moreover assist to reduce ache.

four. Ginger: Research has indicated that ginger has anti-inflammatory outcomes and may aid with ache control. It may be immoderate tremendous to eat ginger tea or add uncooked ginger to meals.

five. Magnesium: This mineral aids in ache treatment and muscular rest. Dark leafy vegetables, nuts, seeds, and complete grains are meals excessive in magnesium.

It is giant to do not forget that dietary strategies should be utilised together with scientific treatments and with a healthcare agency's supervision.

Chapter 11: A Journey Through Time

Identification ancient civilizations additionally struggled with neck ache? Neck ache is not any stranger to humans. Generation upon technology has struggled with pain inside the neck and backbone; however we however deal with it these days. Why is that? How have our strategies of managing neck ache modified in assessment to those in the beyond? Before we get began out on our adventure to resolving neck ache, allows test the ancient thoughts-set on neck pain, including ways remedies have evolved. This will motive a deeper appreciation of modern-day remedy alternatives and knowledge of why treatment is wherein it's far these days.

ANCIENT ACCOUNTS OF NECK PAIN AND REMEDIES

The notable bills that we've got had been given of historic pain control come from the historic civilizations and their experience of continual ache. Chronic pain refers to sustained ache in single or extra common areas over a long term body, commonly as a minimum more than three to six months. Today, continual ache may be almost without problem controlled, thanks to fashionable treatment, which makes it tough for us to understand definitely how chronic ache changed into controlled in ancient times. Let's discover how historic civilizations dealt with neck pain and associated treatments.

First, it is crucial to apprehend what sort of accidents and chronic pain grow to be sustained with the useful useful resource of those in historical times. According to a few belongings, individuals who show arrows the use of a longbow may frequently pull 70 or greater pounds of weight, all the use of the identical positions and gestures (admin, 2020). This has delivered on ordinary accidents that has been the trouble of masses archaeological investigation. This announcement shows the presence of persistent lower back, neck, and shoulder pain, as well as injuries regular with bone spurs.

When it involves historical treatment options, debts variety. It changed into vital for ancient civilizations to apprehend pain control and remedy—of route it grow to be, how might also need to anyone live with such painful injuries continuously? As a cease stop result, the property that have been often to be had—along with vegetation and flowers—have become medicinal. However, in spite of the way not unusual those strategies were in historical instances, the debts in their efficacy variety. Something else that ancient records has communicated to us is that persistent pain, in its numerous forms, has withstood the take a look at of time, impacting us as human beings for millennia.

In special respects, some techniques of curing or alleviating continual neck ache have sustained, proving effective even these days. These strategies commonly encompass stretches and massages that originate from ancient China, surviving through to nowadays. Of path, it makes experience that stretches, an ancient method of bodily treatment in a few respects, have been more effective than rubbing salves at the pores and skin.

Let's soar beforehand a bit in time now. You are in all likelihood acquainted with the present day-day opioid catastrophe, as maximum human beings are. But did you apprehend that the opioid catastrophe has its origins even earlier, as early on as the 20th century? The addictive drug has no longer lost its popularity through the years, because of the reality that, unluckily in loads of respects, opioids are immensely beneficial. During the civil warfare, morphine and similar medicinal tablets had been allowed as remedies for intense injuries, and at one issue within the overdue Nineties, heroin became even considered to be a suitable treatment method for ache.

Just a few a few years later in the mid-twentieth century, some thing referred to as "nerve blockading clinics" sprouted forth. Intended to manipulate pain, the ones clinics served to help manage the impact of continual pain with out strategies as invasive as surgical treatment. It have become no longer until the 70s that human beings have become aware about the effect that these remedies had had; on the same time as they have been effective at treating ache, what changed into going to deal with the myriad of latest signs and signs that those techniques brought about?

And now, we come to these days. Modern day has talented us with such pretty some advantages with reference to treating neck and spinal ache that it is nearly unreal. With the data and experimentation of preceding generations in the back of us, we've got got advanced extra effective strategies which can show to be lifesaving almost approximately the treatment of neck pain. We furthermore have greater effective outlooks on persistent ache manipulate than ever in advance than, making it compellingly obvious that we're at every benefit to cope with continual pain.

"If that is the case, then why am I in pain?" you will be asking.

It boils all the way all of the manner all the way down to a loss of records regarding the ones remedy options, this is one barrier I want to break down close to the remedy of continual neck ache. Throughout this e-book, you could uncover some of the best strategies for treating neck pain that during reality have no longer been accessible to the common man or woman. Now, the ones methods are to be had, and they'll redesign lives—your life.

THE EVOLUTION OF NECK PAIN TREATMENT

Over time, it is going with out pronouncing that the way pain modified into perceived and dealt with has modified drastically over time. The remedy alternatives to be had, especially those touted because the high-quality, have advanced dramatically, which you will be able to see on the timeline underneath. A precise gain of this type of wealthy facts, regardless of the fact that it method pain went untreated for centuries, is that we now apprehend a plethora of strategies that do and do now not paintings.

Pain Management Timeline

If you are inquisitive about facts the information and evolution of pain remedy, and the way we recognize what we understand nowadays, then test this pain manage timeline eventually of statistics (Pain Management History Time Line, n.D.):

1500-1300 BCE.

We start the journey with historical civilizations. At this time, there had been a few beliefs and practices accessible. First, it changed into believed that any ache outdoor of an externally seen harm changed into the paintings of evil spirits. This makes awesome sense due to the predominantly non secular way of lifestyles of the time. At the equal time, Pre-Incan cultures commenced out to apply the leaves of the coca plant for ache manipulate, and opium have grow to be used for ache sooner or later of Egypt, China, India, and special cultures nearby.

460-four hundred BCE.

During this time period—the classical period—pain end up seemed to be the end cease result of a stability some of the 4 humors. The 4 humors were stated to be precise bodily fluids. It become at some stage in this time that Hippocrates stated the usefulness of opium for treating pain. Around 4 hundred BCE got here a few further upgrades, a number of which we but use in recent times. Moving faraway from opium and mandrake remedies, hot and bloodless temperature remedies have been popularized, further to bloodletting and the software program of natural remedies for ache.

3 hundred BCE.

This changed into the early imperial technology. It come to be at some point of this time that it modified into believed that the coronary heart modified into responsible for sensing ache, no longer the brain. This is also at the same time as acupuncture made its first appearance in Chinese clinical texts as a ache consolation technique.

50 CE.

This time period represents past due antiquity, wherein we ultimately understood that the important frightened tool may additionally moreover want to stumble on ache. It have emerge as believed that pain indicated an underlying sickness that need to be handled. Also during this time, the Greeks, Romans, and Egyptians made use of electrical fish for some commonplace pains, alongside side headaches and arthritis.

1150 CE.

Welcome to the Middle Ages. During this period in time, many believed that pain have turn out to be a punishment from the gods, and as a cease end result, us mortals had to heal it. Nikolaus of Salerno wrote the number one e-book of drug recipes in some unspecified time in the future of this time, and it's miles exciting to have a have a look at that greater than 1/2 of the recipes characteristic ache remedies.

1200-1300 CE.

This is at the same time as the number one documented use of narcotic painkillers for painful surgical strategies became added. It is form of appalling to recognize that previous to this, maximum human beings had no ache control alternatives for invasive surgical tactics!

1350 CE.

This became at some level inside the age of exploration, and maximum of the human beings inside the Western worldwide taken into consideration Eastern pain manipulate alternatives as derived from the satan. In Europe, narcotics had been nonetheless all the rage; they often combined them with herbs to area onto sponges, which have been then inhaled or carried out to wounds.

1670s.

This age represents the renaissance and enlightenment, in which pain grow to be taken into consideration as inevitable and a signal that one is residing (pretty philosophical, isn't it?). In this decade, Willem ten Rhijne, a Dutch scientific clinical health practitioner, grow to be the number one Western practitioner to analyze the art work of acupuncture.

1680.

Thomas Sydenham brought a mixture of opium and liquor for ache manipulate.

1683.

Rhijne, the Dutch physician from earlier, posted a quite famous essay on the sensible applications of acupuncture for ache control.

1820-1830.

Quite a bounce from out ultimate length, the late business generation introduced approximately the concept that pain may be controlled or relieved. During this time, Germany and the us started out to industrially produce morphine, a ache manage drug.

1846.

Dentist William T.G. Morton became the primary to offer a public demonstration at the sensible makes use of of ether as a surgical anesthetic. Ether grow to be generally inhaled via patients to render them unconscious at some point of surgical treatment.

1848.

Just years later, British obstetrician James Young Simpson proposed that chloroform be used as a ache remedy for those in childbirth.

1870s.

Just over a long term later, diagnostic assessments had been advanced for sure pain-associated issues. It have end up additionally for the duration of this time that continual ache modified into omitted as a sign of highbrow infection and that medical doctors started out to become worried approximately whether or not or now not or not morphine became addictive (spoiler alert: The solution is positive).

1920s.

During this age, persistent pain was regularly misunderstood and left out, each because the affected individual being delusional or searching for drugs. Psychotherapy or neurosurgery were the maximum exceptionally endorsed alternatives for ache relief proper now.

1947.

William Livingston installed a pain sanatorium inside the United States.

1953.

Dr. John Bonica published The Management of Pain, which served due to the fact the first complete textbook on ache control alternatives international.

1965.

By this time, ache modified into understood as each a mental and physiological hassle. Ronald Melzack and Patrick D. Wall brought some issue referred to as the "gate manage principle of pain," which stimulated how physicians have been capable of assist and talk ache with sufferers.

1970.

Operant conditioning and precise psychological techniques had been considered for pain manipulate.

Nineties.

At the begin of the records era, ache became finally identified as individualized, this means that that every affected individual would should get preserve of a completely unique treatment plan and that greater research revolving round pain may be important. In this decade, it became recognized that pharmacology was no longer sufficient; we needed more techniques for ache manage.

As you could see, there is a lot of facts revolving at some point of the remedy of pain in desired, which furthermore extends to the treatment of neck ache. It is probably beautiful to you the way outlandish a number of the ideals revolving round ache were, but may want to you agree with that many humans hold further superb views on neck pain nowadays? Let's talk about it!

Chapter 12: Understanding The Anatomy Of The Neck And Spine

You understand how so that it will construct a house effectively; you must have a strong foundation? Otherwise, all your hard paintings will come crumbling down round you, causing wasted time, pain, and frustration. Well, your frame is sort of like a house, in that without a robust basis, you cannot assume your body to be satisfied and healthful. And what serves as the foundation for your frame? The neck and resolution, of direction! Carrying out such a number of crucial physical skills, the neck and backbone are chargeable for plenty. Without ensuring that that basis is strong, your fitness is sure to go through.

That's in which expertise the anatomy of the neck and resolution come into play. Without a sturdy basis, you can't have a sturdy house. At one component, I too underestimated just how vital know-how the anatomy of the neck and determination are. However, nowadays, you may recognize the anatomy of each the neck and the backbone. Do now not worry; it will all be defined in easy terms, and I promise you will no longer be bored or burdened. This information lays the muse for later chapters, so buckle up!

THE STRUCTURE OF THE NECK AND ITS FUNCTION

Let's start off smooth—what is the neck? You may have a super definition of the neck than what's elegant, so permit's refine it. According to Britannica, the neck is the part of the body that connects the top on your shoulders and your chest. Some key talents of the neck encompass the seven vertebrae that compose it, the spinal cord, numerous veins and arteries, and different muscle organizations and components that assist you characteristic in a huge number of processes. Neck anatomy can be puzzling, so we are going to spend a while going over it.

Muscles inside the Neck

Did that there are extra than 20 muscle mass within the neck (Neck Muscles: Anatomy, Common Conditions & Disorders, n.D.)? The muscle agencies indoors your neck are so critical because of the truth they allow for vital abilties of lifestyles; for example, even as the muscle mass in your neck are capable of increase and settlement, you are able to reveal your head and carry out movements akin to that. There are many physical talents that make the neck muscular tissues essential to preserve existence. Just a number of the blessings we have got thanks to neck muscle tissues encompass:

Ensuring that you can chew and swallow meals.

Carrying out the motions of speakme.

Helping us to breathe.

Allowing us to move our neck and shoulders.

Supporting our head.

Facilitating sure facial expressions.

And it is just scratching the ground. The muscle tissues for your neck take a look at an complicated form, lining the the front, lower again, and elements of it. There are, generally speakme, 3 agencies of muscle companies inside the neck: Anterior (the front), posterior (again), and lateral (issue).

There are six vital anterior muscle tissues within the neck. The first of the anterior neck muscle mass is the platysma, that could be a thin layer of muscle located within the shoulder and chest place, in addition to the jaw. This muscle in particular is accountable for supporting your jaw circulate and maintaining the pores and skin for your face and neck in location. Then, there can be the sternocleidomastoid, that is one in each of the maximum important muscle agencies which you have in your neck! This muscle allows you to transport your head and neck, further to govern the joint that permits you to open and close your jaw. Another anterior muscle is the subclavius, which lets you drift your shoulders and collar bones. There also are the infrahyoid and scalene muscle tissues. The infrahyoid muscle tissues are in reality four muscle mass that allow you to talk, and the scalene are 3 muscle mass that push your rib cage down so that you can breathe. Every unmarried this kind of muscle groups is important a remarkable manner to be alive.

Next, we've got were given the posterior muscle groups, which might be found within the back of the neck and are further as important. The splenius capitis and splenius cervicis are muscle tissues standard like straps that facilitate the extension and rotation of your head. In addition, the 4 suboccipital muscle tissue are determined at the lowest of the cranium. These muscular tissues are those answerable for how you may flow into your head in dozens of numerous recommendations. There also are transversospinalis muscle groups, which may be 5 muscle groups that allow you to circulate your head in all guidelines as well.

Finally, there are the lateral neck muscle tissues. The rectus capitis anterior and rectus capitis lateralis are   muscle corporations chargeable for helping you flow your neck from the lowest of the top, and the longus capitis and longus colli let you swivel your head.

Neck Compartments

Also called "neck areas," there are four neck cubicles which might be used to consult the contents of the neck. Simply positioned, every compartment holds one-of-a-type elements of your neck. For instance, there can be the vertebral compartment, which incorporates cervical vertebrae and postural muscle tissue. The visceral compartment is wherein your glands lie—including the thyroid—further to the trachea, larynx, and pharynx. Then, there are booths referred to as "vascular booths," which comprise the vagus nerve, jugular vein, and carotid artery, and are determined on every sides of the neck.

From a natural angle, the muscles within the neck and the cubicles are closely intertwined. As you can inform, those elements of the body are very important. The lucky records is that they're blanketed very well. In reality, the booths of the neck are included with the resource of those neck muscle mass we said earlier, this is why muscle damage regularly comes before lifestyles-threatening neck or spinal accidents.

Neck Triangles

There are some more factors of the neck you have to understand about. Namely, we've got the neck triangles. These are triangles which are probably bordered with the aid of the usage of the use of the muscle groups in the neck, and there are two: Anterior and posterior. As you could bet, the ones triangles are positioned at the back and front of the neck respectively. This is absolutely a few other manners that the zones of the neck are categorized and damaged down.

As you could see, there are a whole lot of 1-of-a-kind additives of the neck to apprehend. However, the neck isn't an isolated frame difficulty; other areas of the frame impact the neck as well, that is why it is crucial to check surrounding regions of your body shape.

OVERVIEW OF THE CERVICAL SPINE AND VERTEBRAE

Another vital detail of the health of the neck you want to remember is that of the cervical backbone. The cervical spine starts off evolved its journey within the frame at the bottom of the skull and capabilities itself right proper all the way down to something referred to as the "thoracic spine." The cervical spine helps be a part of the pinnacle to the neck and limbs and serves as a mediator amongst all of these factors of the frame. There are many one-of-a-kind components of the cervical backbone to hold in thoughts, which includes the fact that it isn't always regularly protected, consequently serving as a component of vulnerability at the frame. Otherwise, that allows you to begin your neck ache restoration journey, you need to furthermore recognize approximately the composition of the cervical spine.

The Bony Structure of the Neck

We begin our know-how of cervical backbone composition with a discussion of the neck's bony structure. There are seven cervical vertebrae that incorporate the cervical spine, which range from C1 to C7 in name. The cervical spine moreover consists of the hyoid bone, manubrium of sternum, and clavicles (collar bones). In addition, it is also interesting to recognize that the cervical backbone takes the form of the letter 'C.' This curve, known as the "lordotic curve," is split into additives. The advanced institution is made of vertebrae C1 and C2, on the equal time as the inferior enterprise enterprise is product of the final vertebrae.

Something some of people do now not apprehend about the anatomy of the cervical backbone is that there are in reality joints amongst every of the vertebrae. These joints permit your spine to benefit movement, however the fact that a great deal less movement that we commonly expect from joints like the knees, as an example. Instead, the joints among the ones vertebrae permit for useful crowning glory of one another, facilitating moves like moving your head spherical. There are maximum crucial joints proper proper right here to keep in mind: The atlanto-occipital joint, which lets in us to nod, and the atlanto-axial joint, it absolutely is made from numerous, smaller joints.

This bony form of the neck, at the same time as protected to an extent, is surely one of the more inclined factors of the neck and spinal device. Damage to the cervical spine can be a ways much less tough to preserve than harm to the neck itself in quite a few times, it is why know-how the anatomy of the neck is vital; it allows you to apprehend why your pain is gift and wherein to intention close to resolving that ache. Now, we're going to check the ligaments in the cervical spine.

www.ingramcontent.com/pod-product-compliance
Lightning Source LLC
Chambersburg PA
CBHW060222030426
42335CB00014B/1304